T0187985

Paediatric Surgery

Paediatric surgeons who practice in areas where medical resources are stretched over wide geographical areas face a number of challenges. This resource provides an easy and useful guide to help readers understand the essentials of paediatric surgery. Using the authors' own experiences, the text illustrates the different management practices required when dealing with paediatric patients in rural and remote settings.

The most frequently encountered fetal, infant and paediatric conditions are reviewed, together with coverage of trauma, burns, urology, thoracic surgery, emergency abdominal surgery, minimally invasive paediatric surgery and problems with external genitalia.

This book is intended to be a practical guide for clinicians to the common and important problems seen in paediatric surgery, enabling them to make clinical management plans and ensure effective communication with local teams.

Paediatric Surgery
Clinical Practice in Remote and Rural Settings, and in Tropical Regions

Edited by
Daniel Carroll
Harry Stalewski
Bhanu Mariyappa Rathnamma

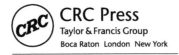

CRC Press
Taylor & Francis Group
Boca Raton London New York

CRC Press is an imprint of the
Taylor & Francis Group, an **informa** business

Cover image: A view of Castle Hill from Queens Gardens in Townsville, Queensland, Australia (Shutterstock 621604079.)

First edition published 2023
by CRC Press
6000 Broken Sound Parkway NW, Suite 300, Boca Raton, FL 33487-2742

and by CRC Press
4 Park Square, Milton Park, Abingdon, Oxon, OX14 4RN

CRC Press is an imprint of Taylor & Francis Group, LLC

ISBN: 9780367742232 (hbk)
ISBN: 9780367713058 (pbk)
ISBN: 9781003156659 (ebk)

DOI: 10.1201/9781003156659

Typeset in Times LT Std
by KnowledgeWorks Global Ltd.

Contents

Preface

My original intention several years ago was to try and distill the knowledge and combined experience of paediatric surgery in the tropics by the team here in Townsville. It was certainly very different to the practice I had experienced in major centres in the UK and Australia, and I could see that there was a definite need to provide insights into some of the differences in practice. Over the prolonged period of writing the book, it has evolved to outline some of the commoner problems we face, not only in the different spectrum of diseases that we encounter but also to include some of the problems relating to remoteness and the social disadvantage among the population that we service.

Writing has been interrupted by serious floods and weather events as well as the COVID pandemic, but throughout we have managed to maintain and expand our service in paediatric surgery. I am immensely grateful for all my colleagues in Townsville and, in particular, Harry and Bhanu and our registrars (particularly Helen Buschel) without who this book would never have happened. The list of people to thank is too large to include in this preface, but it would be remiss of me not to mention our families who have put up with us preparing work for book chapters. I would also like to offer sincere thanks to our nursing and allied health colleagues who probably unknowingly have made several important contributions to my own practice over the last decade. The support of the team at CRC Press/Taylor & Francis (in particular their support of my cavalier attitude to deadlines) has also been essential in allowing this book to grow. Finally, but perhaps most importantly, I think it is important to acknowledge my patients and their families who have been the greatest teachers of all. It has been a privilege and a pleasure to look after them.

Daniel Carroll

Editors

Dr Daniel Carroll went to medical school in Oxford and trained in paediatric surgery and urology in the UK and Australia until becoming a consultant in Cambridge in 2008, where he was the Surgical Lead for Fetal Medicine and held teaching positions both in the hospital where he was in charge of paediatric surgical training and the university. Looking for new challenges, he moved to Tropical North Queensland in 2012 where he became the Director of Paediatric Surgery for North Queensland. He holds a higher degree from Oxford University for research into necrotizing enterocolitis and is an Associate Professor at James Cook University.

Dr Harry Stalewski is an Associate Professor in Clinical Surgery at James Cook University in Queensland. He held multiple roles at the Royal Brisbane Hospital from 1977 to 1981, completing his FRACS II in 1984. Dr Stalewski was a Senior Paediatric Surgery Registrar at both Adelaide Children's Hospital and Queen Elizabeth Hospital for Sick Children, London, before relocating to Townsville in 1987. Since then, he has held a number of board memberships and has chaired both Paediatric Surgery Queensland and the Surgical Specialities Group at Mater Hospital in Townsville.

Dr Bhanu Mariyappa Rathnamma was trained in India, New Zealand and Australia. He obtained a fellowship in paediatric surgery in 2014 and has been working as Consultant Paediatric Surgeon at Townsville University Hospital since 2015. He is a keen teacher and holds the position of Senior Lecturer at James Cook University.

Contributors

Helen Buschel
Paediatric Surgery Registrar
Townsville University Hospital
Townsville, Australia

Michael Thomas Carroll
Economist
Queensland Treasury
Australia

Kyle Crowley
Principal House Officer
Paediatric Surgery
Townsville University Hospital
Townsville, Australia

David Kanaganayangam
Principal House Officer
Paediatric Surgery
Townsville University Hospital
Townsville, Australia

Phoebe Leung
Unaccredited Paediatric Surgery Registrar
Townsville Hospital
Townsville, Australia

Yin Mar Oo
Paediatric Surgeon
Yangon Children's Hospital
Myanmar

Elizabeth McLeod
Paediatric Surgeon
Monash Children's Hospital
Australia

Ramesh Mark Nataraja
Paediatric Surgeon
Monash Children's Simulation & Monash
    Children's Hospital
Australia

Kapilan Ravichandran
Surgical Registrar (PHO)
Townsville University Hospital
Townsville, Australia

Kiera Roberts
Paediatric Surgery Trainee
Women's and Children's Hospital
Adelaide, Australia

Charlotte Julia Slaney
Consultant Radiologist
Queensland X-Ray
Townsville, Australia

The Tropics

1

Michael Thomas Carroll and Daniel Carroll

The tropics, or equatorial regions, for centuries have stirred interest among people living outside of the region. Old Western literature often represented the tropics as a wild, unconquerable natural wilderness, or as "Garden of Eden" style tropic paradise. Twentieth-century Western scholars viewed the region as relatively more inhospitable towards human civilisation than the colder climates of Europe and North America, suggesting that the humid, hot climates of the equatorial regions correlate to the human populations being unable to gain control over nature.

Whilst Western literature might have exaggerated the tropics wildness and inhospitality, it is markedly hotter, wetter, and more humid than temperate regions of the planet. Additionally, the region experiences much higher levels of extreme weather, including regular tropical cyclones, monsoonal flooding, and severe thunderstorms. Despite this, the equatorial region is home to a rapidly growing population, currently 3.3 billion people live in the tropics, representing over 40% of the world's population, and the region is expected to host more than half of the Earth's population by 2050.

According to the geographic definition, the tropics are the regions of Earth surrounding the equator between the lines of the Tropic of Cancer in the Northern Hemisphere and the tropic of Capricorn in the Southern Hemisphere, including all zones on Earth where the Sun contacts a point directly overhead. This region is illustrated in Figure 1.1, encompassing large areas of sub-Saharan Africa, southern India, South-East Asia, Oceania, South and Central America, and Northern Australia. Within the tropics are the majority of the least developed countries (LDCs), all of which experience high levels of poverty, human resource weakness, and economic vulnerability, with almost 670 million living in extreme poverty in 2019.

Despite the technical definition, the conditions experienced within the equatorial zone are rapidly expanding poleward as a result of climate change, with the American Geophysical Union calculating in 2020 the expansion of the tropical zone to be between 27.75 and 55.5 kilometres every ten years. Consequently, the climatic conditions and extreme weather events experienced in the tropics are becoming more and more prevalent in the middle latitudes of the Earth.

Understanding the health challenges experienced within the tropics is becoming ever more relevant and important in a modern, globalised Earth. This is a result of rapid population growth being experienced within the region, as well as ongoing poleward expansion of the equatorial region.

CLIMATE AND WEATHER

Tropical Climate

Throughout the tropics, there is a range of different climate biomes present. However, most regions in the tropics experience warm to hot temperatures all year round, with high levels of humidity.

DOI: 10.1201/9781003156659-1

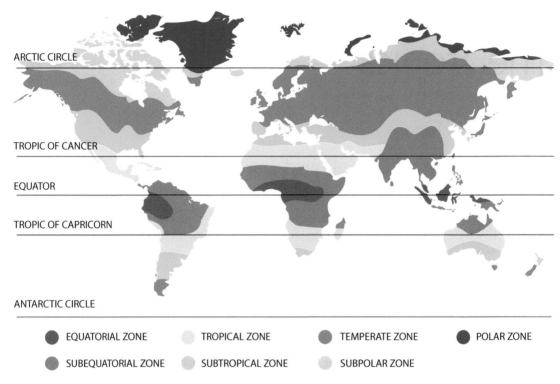

FIGURE 1.1   World map showing areas within the Tropics. (Shutterstock image 1445255762.)

Most inhabited tropical areas have a wet season and a dry season, experiencing a monsoon trough in the warmer summer months. During this wet season, there are often daily showers, with constantly high humidity levels. Additionally, during the wet season, air and water quality improve, and vegetation experiences significant growth, raising crop yields towards the end of the season. However, the wet season also regularly results in widespread flooding, causing the destruction of natural and human infrastructure, erosion increases, and soil nutrients can be diminished. The wet season also corresponds with the increased incidence of several insect-borne diseases such as malaria, as well as other infectious diseases such as melioidosis. Biomes that have a monsoonal wet season include seasonal forests and savannahs.

Tropical rainforests are also widespread within the geographical tropics; however, they do not experience wet and dry seasons, having equally distributed rainfall throughout the year, being consistently wet, humid, and warm.

Regions within the tropics do not necessarily have a tropical climate, with much of the area of the equatorial zone being arid or semi-arid, including the Australian Outback, the Atacama Desert, and the Sahara Desert. Additionally, there are isolated instances of alpine tundra, such as the Carstensz Glacier in New Guinea, and the Andes Mountains in Chile and Peru.

Tropical Weather

The tropical latitudes correspond to higher incidences of extreme weather, including tropical cyclones, thunderstorms, and tornadoes. Much of this extreme weather occurs during the wet season with the monsoon.

Tropical cyclones, also referred to as hurricanes or typhoons, are the most intense form of extreme weather within the tropics. They form as a result of warm ocean waters and regularly make landfall along tropical coastlines during the warmer wet season months. They can cause significant damage, especially to coastal regions, contributing to storm surges, severe thunderstorms, high winds, spawning tornadoes, and high levels of precipitation. Tropical cyclones often result in widespread flooding and have massive human impacts, resulting in thousands of deaths. For example, the 1970 Bhola cyclone was responsible for the deaths of over 500,000 people, primarily in the Ganges Delta region of Bangladesh. Additionally, cyclones can result in billions of dollars of damage even after weakening, such as in 1975, when ex-Typhoon Nina brought heavy rainfall and flooding to the Henan Province of China, leading to the collapse of the Banqiao Dam and the death of 100,000 people.

Tropical cyclones are regular contributors to widespread damage and can cause extensive flooding. Monsoon troughs often bring devastating levels of precipitation to the tropics during the wet season without any example of extreme weather. In January 2019, a tropical low became embedded within a stalled, a vigorously active monsoonal trough between Townsville and Mt Isa, dropping thousands of millimetres of rainfall over 2 weeks with little movement or respite. The result was floods submerging 25,000 square kilometres, creating an inland sea in Queensland, roughly an area the size of Belgium.

The Subtropics, the Expanding Equatorial Zone, and Climate Change

Outside of the tropics, monsoonal troughs are also widespread through parts of the subtropics, with tropical cyclones regularly impacting regions in the higher latitudes, or converting to extratropical cyclones. A notable example of extreme tropical weather impacting the subtropics is Hurricane Katrina, which in 2005 tracked over New Orleans, Louisiana, killing over 1,800 people and wrecking over $US125 billion in damage.

The effects of tropical cyclones and monsoonal troughs are expected to be experienced in higher and higher latitudes over the coming century, as the equatorial zone tracks rapidly northwards. Consequently, millions more will be placed at higher risk of the effects of monsoonal flooding and cyclonic weather.

Additionally, meteorologists suggest that flooding and tropical cyclones within the tropics themselves are becoming more and more intense as climate indicators change. On top of this, droughts in the tropics are becoming more common and elongated. Coupled with the rapidly increasing population in the region, water scarcity is quickly intensifying as a major problem for communities in the tropics.

Additionally, as populations rapidly expand, land degradation is accelerating in the region, with topsoil being removed at an astonishing rate, meaning vital agricultural land is being lost. Desertification is also becoming an increasingly prevalent phenomenon in tropical savannah land in South America and sub-Saharan Africa, as well as across the subtropics. Increased water scarcity, more intense flooding, desertification, and land degradation all pose a massive threat to the billions of people in the tropics and the sustainability of their inhabitation, with both infrastructure and agriculture being threatened by changing climates, posing risks of widespread population displacement and devastating famines.

HUMAN SYSTEMS IN THE TROPICS

The tropics are home to over 3.3 billion people, with its population growing much faster than the rest of the world. By 2050, it will be home to far more than half of the global population. However, the tropics include the majority of the world's LDCs, characterised by poverty, human resource weakness, and extremely vulnerable economic systems. In conjunction with a lack of economic and social development, countries in the tropics are plagued with political instability, often stemming into conflict. Additionally, famine and drought regularly impact tropical populations, an issue becoming more and more prevalent, and populations rapidly increase because of that. Extreme poverty is common and widespread across the equatorial zone, with more than half of the total population living in poverty. On top of, and often exacerbated by, these problems, regions in the tropics are faced with numerous endemic and vexatious health problems which degrade the well-being of the billions living in these regions.

Economics in the Tropics

Economic growth in the tropics has been significantly stunted for several decades, since a debt crisis in the 1980s devastated the economies in many tropical countries, especially in Latin America. Whilst gross domestic product (GDP) per capita increased in the tropics between the 2008 and 2009 global financial crisis (GFC) and the COVID-19 pandemic in 2020, the existing GDP per capita gap between economies in the tropics and those in the rest of the world grew larger, indicating that economic growth in the region has been unable to adapt as quickly as more economically developed regions, meaning those in the tropics are being left behind economically in a globalised world.

Many countries in the tropics, especially in sub-Saharan Africa, score highly on the economic vulnerability index, a criterion used by the United Nations to identify LDCs. This index describes a country's exposure and vulnerability to economic weakness as a result of localised or globalised disruptions to normal economic activities. In particular, LDCs are especially vulnerable to interruptions in export and import services. As such, these developing economies are highly receptive to globalised downturns, such as the 2008–2009 GFC and the COVID-19 pandemic, and are often disproportionately affected by such economic crises. Additionally, LDCs are often highly reliant on agricultural industries, which are often vulnerable to natural disasters. As such, an increased prevalence of extreme weather events such as drought and cyclones as a result of climate change threatens the economic stability of many countries in the tropics.

Many economies in the tropics have high levels of debt, which has been a persistent problem for governments in the region for decades. The 1980–1990 Latin American debt crisis saw real wage drops of upto 40%, as well as skyrocketing prices, large-scale unemployment, and GDP per capita growth rate of almost −9% across Latin America over five years. Most extremely, in Argentina, stagflation as a result of defaults meant the country had to adopt a new currency in order to avoid complete economic collapse. Since 2008–2009, GFC debt levels and services in the tropics have increased significantly, and currently all but one heavily indebted poor country is in the tropics. These increasing debt levels signal possible future debt challenges in the tropics, especially in LDCs, which could result in a prolonged recession, as happened in the Latin American debt crisis, and severely impact the future sustainability of the tropical countries.

Another key feature in many tropical economies is the level of remittances being received. As of 2017 remittances accounted for approximately 2.3% of the total tropical GDP, compared to just over 1% of the total global GDP. Remittances account for over 10% of the GDP in several tropical countries, including the Philippines, Haiti, and the Gambia, and remittances made up 39% of the GDP in Tonga in 2019. Pacific Island nations are particularly dependent on remittances, with countries such as Kiribati, Samoa, and Tonga being completely reliant on remittances and foreign aid.

Economic development is strongly correlated to violent conflict, with many tropical countries, especially LDCs, caught in a "conflict trap". Conflict lowers income and economic activity in a country; as physical capital is destroyed, resources are diverted to military spending, divestment, and exchange disruption. Recovery from a conflict is uneven and unsure, and often conflict resumes after a short period of respite, hampering any economic sustainability. Examples of this include Angola, Guinea-Bissau, and Liberia.

Geopolitical Instability in the Tropics

Poverty and the tropics

Despite consistent improvements in global poverty levels, there remains a major issue across the tropics, with approximately 60% of the total population living in extreme or moderate poverty. The region accounts for 85% of world's population living in extreme poverty, with 50% of the extreme poor living in just five tropical countries – Nigeria, the Democratic Republic of the Congo, Ethiopia, India, and Bangladesh. Even more concerningly, the number of people living in moderate poverty in the tropics increased from 2014 to 2020, numbering more than 1.3 billion.

A common characteristic of extreme poverty is undernourishment. Throughout the 20th century, undernourishment rates in the tropics consistently decreased; however, there has been a recent reversal in this trend, with more than 800 million people suffering from undernourishment worldwide. Notably, climate change is expected to contribute significantly towards increased water scarcity and desertification, placing millions of hectares of arable land at threat. This is coupled with an increasing prevalence of destructive weather events such as tropical cyclones. These changing climate indicators pose a major risk to the food security of millions, increasing the risk of devastating famines and an increase in the prevalence of undernourishment, especially in sub-Saharan Africa. Additionally, political and economic instability in many regions of the tropics contributes to increased undernourishment, with wars across the region displacing millions and resulting in massive crop losses annually.

Health in the tropics

Undernourishment and malnutrition are particularly prevalent in children under the age of five and result in lifelong impacts, stunting physical and mental growth, and contributing to about one-third of all deaths in children.

Despite the predicted rise in the population of this area, there is a relative lack of paediatric surgical services when compared to other areas. There are well-known inequities in healthcare provision between developing and developed nations. Even within developed nations like Australia, there are striking health inequalities between different groups, with the worst health outcomes being seen in the indigenous population. A larger proportion of indigenous people (Aboriginal and Torres Strait Islanders) still live in tropical areas of Australia.

Our practice in North Queensland encompasses a large area of both tropical and subtropical areas, exhibiting a climate ranging from dry to wet subtropical areas. There are large areas of sparsely populated arid areas away from the coast in the West of our region and major population centres are congregated around the larger towns along the Eastern coast. In the North of the region, there are rainforests which meet the sea in places, and in the South of the region, there are dry subtropical areas. We are subject to two major seasons, the wet monsoonal period during the summer months and a dry period during the Australian winter. The weather is often unpredictable in the wet season and we are subject to major weather events with cyclones and flooding at this time. These extreme weather events are becoming more frequent and often impact our ability to transport patients around the region.

We are fortunate to be part of a developed healthcare system, offering tertiary-level paediatric surgery, and are one of the few paediatric surgical centres in the world located in the tropics. We provide services to patients from Treaty villages in Papua New Guinea in the North, to the Island communities of the Torres Strait, as well as meeting the paediatric surgical needs of patients in the remote and rural areas of North-West Queensland. We see a variety of paediatric surgical conditions, and the pattern of disease and the presentation are somewhat different to that seen in major metropolitan areas. We see an increased burden of infectious diseases affecting our population, and the surgical management of these problems is an important part of our practice.

The future

As populations continue to rise in the tropics, we will see an increasing number of patients seeking paediatric surgical services. The WHO has identified access to surgery as a key target for improvement in global health. In addition to the increasing population in the tropics, we also see more children as an overall percentage of the population and so the provision of paediatric surgical services will be essential to improving healthcare outcomes for the population overall. The impact of climate change and antimicrobial resistance to antibiotic therapies will become an increasing challenge over time, and we must plan services for the future to meet the needs of our patients and their families. Even within Australia, internal migration into tropical areas has been strong over the last few years with people relocating from major metropolitan centres to smaller cities and regional areas. There is a strong need to anticipate these changes and by tailoring services to meet the needs of the population and the different range of diseases we encounter we can better meet these challenges. New technologies and approaches to medicines such as telemedicine offer great potential to improve outcomes for patients as well as potential efficiencies.

FURTHER READING

American Geophysical Union. "The tropics are expanding, and climate change is the primary culprit." ScienceDaily. ScienceDaily, 18 August 2020. www.sciencedaily.com/releases/2020/08/200818094013.htm.

David Arnold, "Illusory Riches: Representations of the Tropical World, 1840–1950," *Journal of Tropical Geography* 21(1): 6–18, accessed January 6, 2020, doi: 10.1111/1467-9493.00060.

Ian Ridpath ed., *A Dictionary of Astromony* (Oxford: Oxford University Press, 1997).

State of the Tropics (2020). State of the Tropics 2020 Report. James Cook University, Townsville, Australia, 7.

The Tyranny of Distance

2

Daniel Carroll

It is widely accepted that Australia's geographical remoteness has been central in shaping the country's development. It is especially true that geographical isolation of many patients and surgeons from other centres and treatment options will continue to shape the delivery of paediatric surgery to patients living in tropical areas.

In our practice, roughly two-thirds of patients live in areas remote to our tertiary-level referral centre, and treatment options range from simple telephone advice and supported decision-making to urgent aeromedical transfer. In this chapter, we seek to examine the options available to us in a first-world setting with a view to facilitating local expertise and resource utilisation in other settings.

THE HISTORY OF TELEHEALTH

It is remarkable to consider that the first recorded example of the use of the telephone to facilitate medical attention was also the very first recorded example of the use of the telephone. In 1876, when Alexander Graham Bell first successfully used the telephone, it was to get help from his assistant Mr Watson after he spilt sulphuric acid from the wet battery on his trousers (Figure 2.1).

Since then, advances in communication have provided the opportunity to improve medical care to patients geographically removed from healthcare resources. In 1879, the *Lancet* reported a case of a child successfully diagnosed by listening to the nature of the cough to exclude croup. The physician reported the case anonymously but managed to facilitate a three-way consultation with the grandmother and mother and successfully reassured the family that he did not require to visit the child in the middle of the night.

By 1891, other physicians were making repeated reports of the usefulness of the telephone in assisting medical care, and Dr Davy wrote to the *Lancet* proposing that access to beds for patients could be ensured by communicating between hospitals using the telephone. Again, the patient was a child with a broken leg who endured multiple failed attempts at admission to hospital for treatment. It has been clear from the advent of the telephone that advances in telecommunications have been closely followed by attempts to use the new technology to improve patient care.

THE PRESENT

Queensland Health provides telehealth to over 200 different locations throughout our state. The tropical and subtropical areas of far North Queensland cover a vast geographical area (around 800,000 square kilometres), and it is here that telehealth is most of the greatest benefit in assessing and aiding treatment in patients for whom

DOI: 10.1201/9781003156659-2

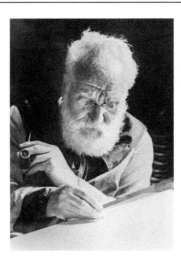

FIGURE 2.1   Alexander Graham Bell. (Shutterstock image 242820268.)

immediate transfer to larger centres is not always practical or possible. We provide telehealth-facilitated outpatient clinic appointments to 100 different centres (33 local hospitals and 67 primary healthcare centres) and offer telehealth-assisted burn advice throughout the Northern half of the state. Our geographical isolation found us well prepared for the COVID global pandemic as we were already familiar with the challenges of delivering care remotely. We use a combination of telephone advice with teleconference facilities to facilitate communication between multiple teams, and video-assisted consultations, with reviewing of pathology results and digital images of patients as well as radiology to assist in decision-making. We have a dedicated secure email service for transfer of images (particularly used for burn assessment) and the larger hospitals in our region share a combined integrated electronic medical record, making it possible to document contemporaneously during consultations.

A variety of free as well as commercially available video solutions are available and, at the moment, we mostly use Cisco Jabber and Queensland Health telehealth software and hardware rather than FaceTime and Skype. The disadvantage of using the dedicated systems is that it requires both the recipient and provider to be in an area where the videoconferencing systems are available, but the quality of communication and stability of the connection are usually excellent. There are obvious advantages to remote consultations, and these include:

- Reduced travel time for patients and their families
- Cultural safety (allowing indigenous communities to remain in their culturally safe environment, with more appropriate local support)
- Reduced risk of travel and introduction of COVID into remote areas and vulnerable communities

It is important, however, to acknowledge that there are limitations to telehealth, as patient contact is reduced, clinical examination is usually more limited, and it is time-consuming for providers with extra costs for equipment and clinic organisation.

Pitfalls and Limitations in Remote Management of Patients

Whilst an enormous amount of information gathering is possible for patients in remote settings, it is important to acknowledge that there are limitations, and that almost always clinical assessment is limited and more time-consuming than when medical consultations are performed face-to-face.

The first and most important component of information gathering relies on a carefully taken, guided history of the problem. Sometimes patients are critically unwell, in which case resuscitation and expeditious transfer to a larger centre are required; however, this is uncommon. In such situations, a clear history of the timing of any injury or onset of symptoms should be ascertained at the same time as initiating resuscitation and transfer.

It is not uncommon for transport considerations to result in a significant delay in transfer, giving the opportunity for a more detailed history to be taken as well as a more detailed assessment of the child and even appropriate investigations to be initiated. In our practice, the most common reason to have to transfer a paediatric surgical patient is because of trauma (including large body surface area [BSA] burns). In such circumstances, it is appropriate to initiate management as per Advanced Paediatric Life Support (APLS) or local guidelines, but it is often helpful for decision-making to be supported by advice from the paediatric surgical team. Teams responsible for aeromedical transfer (such as the Royal Flying Doctor Service [RFDS]) are usually extremely expert in initiating appropriate resuscitation and stabilisation of patients prior to transfer.

Thankfully, for the majority of patients, the situation is not usually critical and often advice and remote management of the problem is possible. For patients with routine or nonemergent presentations, then often telehealth supported consultations are a preferable alternative to face-to-face consultations. The advantages to patients and their families are obvious in that travel time is significantly reduced, and for patients living in remote communities, it is possible to maintain *cultural safety* during consultation, improving engagement with disadvantaged and vulnerable indigenous populations.

Although clinical examination can be performed by proxy with a suitably trained healthcare worker examining the patient on behalf of the surgeon. Unfortunately, despite the opportunities that it presents, we find that certain common conditions are difficult to assess via telehealth. In particular, it has been my experience that the initial assessment of the location and disposition of the testes and abnormalities of the external genitalia are difficult to assess adequately even with the use of digital photography as an adjunct to the telehealth appointment. However, patients can be satisfactorily followed up after routine surgery and after simple emergency procedures (such as trauma, burns, appendectomy) relatively easily. For certain conditions, it is often very straightforward to manage patients remotely, in particular, patients with congenital anomalies of the kidney and urinary tract (CAKUT) requiring regular radiological surveillance – progression of the disease can be managed well via telehealth as often very little extra information is gained by clinical examination in the majority of these patients.

Requirements for Effective Telehealth

- Access to good-quality internet with a stable connection for both the recipient (patient) and provider (paediatric surgeon). Good-quality audio-visual software such as Cisco Jabber is helpful in maintaining a high-quality connection.
- Availability of a suitably trained HCW in the recipient's location to ensure adequate documentation and facilitate access to local resources e.g. dressings, prescription, medical imaging.
- An understanding by the provider of locally available resources and geography.
- Cultural training to meet the needs of vulnerable indigenous populations by providing a culturally safe environment.
- Extra time needs to be allocated to individual patients and time needs to be set aside before clinic visits to gather information and review results.
- Communication and connection difficulties are common, and extra time should be allowed between patients to allow for connection to remote sites.
- Documentation, including follow-up arrangements and communication with wider members of the multidisciplinary team, is essential and written and electronic communication to families and local clinicians.

The Management of Emergency Patients via Telehealth

Over the past decade, we have come to increasingly utilise telehealth as an adjunct to telephone calls to assist in the management of emergency presentations remotely. It is often possible to position work-stations so that the telehealth provider can directly see the patient during the consultation and almost always possible to review radiology and other investigations remotely. This can be particularly useful when no doctor or only relatively junior medical staff are available locally. Guided clinical examination can be helpful, particularly when used in combination with an assessment of vital signs (pulse, blood pressure, temperature).

Management of Trauma via Telehealth

- *History*
  - Time since injury; mechanism of injury; history of subsequent events
- *Examination*
  - Vital signs; urine output; capillary refill time; respiratory rate; pulse oximetry
- *Management of airway/breathing/circulation/cervical spine*
  - Ongoing concomitant resuscitation

It is often useful to use videoconferencing to gain some perspective as to the severity of injuries to allow triage and appropriate resource allocation as an adjunct to telephone advice prior to initiating transfer. Appropriate assessment and initiation of basic treatment, including effective and adequate analgesia often allows for patients' transfer to be organised in the safest and most efficient possible way (both for the patients and their carers/family), as well as reducing demands for scarce resources (aeromedical transfer staff/equipment).

Information Required for Urgent Telehealth Assessment

Although clinical scenarios will vary, it is usually important to gather the following information when providing advice:

- *Patient location*
  - Available local medical resources
  - Available local HCW/medical staff
  - Accessibility (plane/helicopter/4×4/ambulance)
  - Local weather conditions

- *Patient presentation*
  - Nature of illness
  - Suspected diagnosis/problems
  - Duration of illness (often patient presentation can be delayed in remote areas)
- *Previous medical/surgical history*
  - Age
  - Birth weight/antenatal problems
  - Family and social history
- *Family resources/cultural factors*
  - Family members present/available
  - Family situation
  - Consent issues
  - Requirements for social support
  - Need for accommodation for family
  - Needs and support for other children/family members
- *Current management*
  - Last meal/starvation status
  - Fluids administered or proposed
  - Antibiotics given or proposed
  - Analgesia given
  - Medications given
  - Lines (IV access/NGT/catheter/drains)
- *Physical findings*
  - Clinical signs (abdominal signs of peritonitis/obstruction)
  - Respiratory status (including signs of trauma, rib fracture/pneumothorax)
  - Cardiovascular status (including peripheral pulses)
  - Other relevant signs (e.g. BSA burns, limb fractures)
- *Transport considerations*
  - Potential for deterioration
  - Available medical support in flight and pre-flight
  - Safety of transport team
  - Disposition of 'assets' (aircraft/crew)
  - Family support, need for other family members to travel
- *Management prior to transfer*
  - Resuscitation/stabilisation
  - Ongoing communication between different teams throughout process
  - Ensure adequate documentation both locally and in receiving centre
  - Record contact details of involved team members/family
- *Child protection legal issues*
  - If there are concerns around child protection these should be addressed
  - It is important to involve police in some circumstances
- *Post-transfer arrangements*
  - When they arrive at the receiving centre where should they be admitted?
  - Some patients require admission via ED and ongoing assessment
  - Some patients require direct admission to HDU/PICU
  - Some patients can be admitted onto the paediatric ward
  - Some patients are likely to require emergency surgery
  - It is essential to communicate with these teams prior to transfer

COMMUNICATION AND TEAMWORK ARE ESSENTIAL IN SUCCESSFUL MANAGEMENT

Transfers can take many hours and even days in some circumstances, and it is important to revisit the clinical situation, support the local team and update relevant team members if things change over time.

Remote Management Options

There are many different options available for telehealth provision; in Queensland Health we use specifically designed videoconference software which usually affords a stable and secure communication connection between centres. Such systems have the advantage of good-quality connections but require both the provider and the recipient to share software and have appropriately trained team members in both sites available to facilitate its use. This is often less useful and often not available in emergency situations (particularly out of hours). Free videoconferencing alternatives are now widely available such as FaceTime and Skype when videoconferencing facilities are not available, but concerns around data security and stability of connection often limit their usefulness. Usually, a telephone conference call is a useful way of planning patient care, and the following teams are usually required:

- Telehealth recipient (HCW with patient)
- Transport services
- Paediatric surgical team member (usually most senior available team member)
- PICU team member (if required due to severe illness or need for planned admission)
- When necessary other clinicians who may be involved after retrieval (e.g. paediatric team member, neurosurgery team member)

CLINICAL BENEFITS OF TELEHEALTH/REMOTE MANAGEMENT OF PATIENTS

Although it is often time-consuming to create a system to manage patients remotely, there are a number of obvious benefits to both patients and to the healthcare system in making this investment in terms of time, training and equipment to provide this capability.

Benefits to Clinicians/Hospitals

- Earlier institution of effective management of complex problems
- Positive impact on demand for transport requirements
- Collegial support for remote HCWs
- Professional development/training/educational opportunities

Benefits to Patients/Families

- Reduction in need for travel, disruption to family life
- *Cultural safety* for vulnerable populations
- Improve access to healthcare services for remote families
- Reduce patient/family travel costs
- Reduce time away from home for families

THE FUTURE OF TELEHEALTH

As we become ever more connected digitally, it is possible that in the future less travel to regional centres to provide suitable healthcare will be less common. This will be of particular benefit to patients living in remote and rural areas, as at the moment there is a clear healthcare deficit to these patients. As we become more skilled at providing healthcare in this way, both by improving technology and by empowering physicians to learn how best to manage consultations, we will be able to reduce significantly the need for patients to travel long distances for routine appointments. There are obvious advantages in terms of reducing the carbon footprint for healthcare provision, as well as improving convenience and acceptability to patients living in remote areas, who previously have been poorly serviced by healthcare. The key to improvements lies in the following areas:

- Education (both of patients and HCWs as to the availability of telehealth options for treatment)
- Support for remote HCWs (tertiary-level advice to facilitate consultations)
- Collegiality (HCWs feel more confident to manage more difficult cases with appropriate support)
- Improved outcomes for vulnerable patient groups (able to engage more appropriately with Aboriginal and Torres Strait Islander patients who do not wish to travel from their own community)

Other Strategies for Improving Healthcare in Remote Areas

Although we have concentrated on the use of telemedicine to improve access to paediatric surgical services, the strategy within our region is more nuanced. We provide an ***in-reach*** service to larger centres where we travel regularly to other larger hospitals to offer paediatric surgical services. This 'hub and spoke' strategy has been commonplace in medical settings for many years. When done well it is possible to build capacity at a local level by improving clinician engagement with tertiary-level services, offering training opportunities for local teams. It is not practical to offer in-reach services to all centres as a certain volume of patients is required to make it an effective use of clinical time. There are obvious advantages to families reducing travel time and providing care closer to home. These services are central to the strategy from professional bodies such as Royal Australasian College of Surgeons (RACS) in reducing healthcare inequities in regional and remote areas. The expansion of these services lies at the heart of our strategy for improving healthcare outcomes in paediatric surgery in North Queensland. Currently, we offer these services to the Torres Strait, Cairns and Mackay. Unfortunately, these services are limited to the provision of elective care and require significant investment in terms of paediatric surgical time to work because of the extended travel time required (particularly for services to the Torres Strait). Future opportunities to provide increased capacity in these areas are a central component of our longer-term strategy for paediatric surgical services in North Queensland.

SUMMARY

Equity in healthcare for remote and rural patients is a key area for improvement across many countries. Improving access to surgical services will be central to improving healthcare in tropical areas where large distances separating patients from suitable services have previously limited care. The use of new technologies has been accelerated by the global response to the pandemic and appropriate funding and development of services to take account of these advances can play an important part in closing the equity gap to disadvantaged communities.

FURTHER READING

Burke BL Jr. Telemedicine: Pediatric applications. Pediatrics. 2015 July;136(1):e293–e308.
Tully L, et al. Barriers and facilitators for implementing paediatric telemedicine: Rapid review of user perspectives. Front Pediatr. 2021 March;9. Open access Article 630635.

Transport Considerations

3

Daniel Carroll

INTRODUCTION

Although the tropical environment shares many common features between different countries and cultures, one common theme is the relative paucity and undersupply of paediatric surgical services in all of these locations. Because of this, it is often necessary for patients to be transferred long distances to access healthcare services. This is particularly true in Northern Australia, where there is only one paediatric surgical centre in the whole of Northern Australia (above Brisbane). This means that patients often have to be transferred very large distances.

Emergency patient transfers are expensive, sometimes dangerous and always inconvenient for families and patients. It often means that patients undergo deterioration whilst awaiting transport services, and it is important to only transfer patients when definitive care cannot be provided locally with appropriate support. An understanding of the basics of patient transport options is important to appropriately provide care and advice in such settings. Here we will outline the transport options available in North Queensland as well as discuss relevant important considerations when offering clinical advice to patients who need to be transferred to another centre.

WHICH PATIENTS NEED TRANSFER

It is not uncommon for doctors to feel isolated in remote postings, often with few colleagues with whom to discuss cases. In such instances, it is vitally important to try and seek advice as early as possible from receiving teams. **This will not always lead to transfer** and sometimes with appropriate advice it is possible for a patient to be managed remotely using telehealth or transferred electively. However, a small number of paediatric patients require transfer to larger centres for definitive management following acute presentations.

In general, if a transfer is being considered, it is optimal for the most senior clinician available in the referring centre to be involved in facilitating this, often by direct liaison with the accepting surgeon. This reduces the risk of miscommunication and inappropriate management. Once a decision has been made that a patient requires transfer, then it is important to involve transport services/retrieval co-ordinator who are in a position to facilitate a safe transfer and deploy appropriate assets (both personnel and equipment) to allow this to happen. Retrieval teams are often unable to provide an immediate transfer due to resource limitations, and involving them early in the decision-making process is almost always valuable.

DOI: 10.1201/9781003156659-3

It would be impossible to produce an exhaustive list of patients who require transfer to tertiary-level centres with paediatric surgical conditions, but a number of common reasons for aeromedical retrieval are listed as follows:

- Major trauma (particularly with major head injury)
- Major burns (>10%), children under one year of age, specialised areas e.g. genitals, face, airway
- Airway compromise
- Potential for deterioration and lack of surgical paediatric anaesthesia services
- Need for higher-level care e.g. PICU
- Oesophageal foreign bodies e.g. button batteries
- Need for neonatal surgery e.g. possible volvulus, imperforate anus, perforation
- Complicated pneumonia requiring surgical intervention e.g. empyema
- No other transport options e.g. island location
- Need for further investigations not available locally e.g. radiology
- Need for other teams not available locally e.g. vascular surgery, interventional radiology
- Repatriation to usual hospital/team

TYPES OF RETRIEVAL

Retrieval can be subclassified into *primary, secondary* and *tertiary* retrievals. In a primary retrieval, a patient is transferred to an initial hospital. This may either be to their closest hospital or directly to a larger and more appropriately resourced healthcare facility (such as a trauma centre). Secondary retrievals transport a patient from a non-specialised hospital to a hospital where there is a higher level of care available e.g. neuro-surgery, paediatric surgery. Tertiary retrievals transport patients between two similarly specialised hospitals.

Consulting with the Retrieval Co-Ordinator

When contacting another team, it is helpful to be clear and methodical in presentation. This is often helped by writing down your findings first and then applying a structured approach to giving information. Often the assessment locally is entirely correct as you have more information than those receiving the referral. One commonly used structured approach in communicating important clinical information over the telephone is denoted by the acronym ISOBAR and is described in more detail as follows.

ISOBAR-STRUCTURED APPROACH TO TELEPHONE CONSULTATIONS

- **I** **Identify** yourself and identify name and spelling of receiving doctor.
- **S** **Situation** and Status of patient – why are you calling (patient name/suspected diagnosis/ clinical severity of problem)?
- **O** **Observations** most recent vital signs of patient (PR/BP/GCS/PEWS score).
- **B** **Background** history of presenting problems, evaluation, allergies, current medications, treatment given so far.
- **A** **Agree to a plan** I would like advice, orders, evacuation. Agree on level of urgency and agree on a plan of action (e.g. contact retrieval co-ordinator).
- **R** **Recommendations** and **read back** confirm shared understanding of what needs to happen and who is doing what and when, identify parameters for escalation and identify any risks.

Retrieval Services in North Queensland

Retrieval services will be vary in different locations, dependent upon resources. Here we outline the services available in North Queensland as an illustration of how a retrieval service can be delivered.

Even if the need for patient transport has not been confirmed, it is useful to contact the retrieval service early to allow for appropriate allocation of resources. For most larger services, retrievals are co-ordinated by **Retrieval Services Queensland (RSQ)**.

For some smaller centres, it is usual to contact Royal Flying Doctor Service (RFDS) first who will liaise directly with RSQ. It is important to keep retrieval services updated if there are any significant changes in clinical condition as it may be possible to change the flight priority.

Retrieval Services Queensland

RSQ provides clinical co-ordination for aeromedical transfer of patients across North Queensland, including the Torres Strait. They utilise multiple government and non-government organisations to achieve aeromedical coverage of Queensland, including the RFDS and Queensland Ambulance Service (QAS), QG Air Helicopter Rescue and Life Flight Retrieval Medicine. They provide specialist medical and nursing co-ordinators for adult, paediatric neonatal and high-risk obstetrics patients (see Figure 3.1).

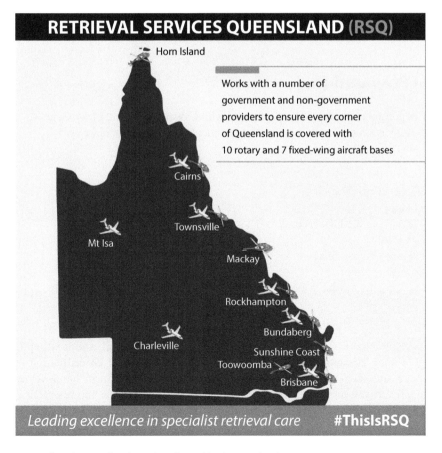

FIGURE 3.1 Map showing retrieval services based in Queensland.

Once retrieval services have been contacted, then it is usually possible to implement a multidisciplinary consultation with important stakeholders being involved in the discussions around management of the patient. Practically what this entails is opening a telephone consultation where the paediatric surgical consultant, referring team and retrieval services co-ordinator are a party to the discussions surrounding immediate and short-term management. These conversations can also involve other teams as necessary, particularly paediatricians and PICU or NICU teams. Occasionally, teams such as radiology or other surgical teams may be necessary to gain further advice about availability of specialised services.

The following paediatric patients should be discussed with RSQ:

- Patients with major trauma or burns
- Patients requiring aeromedical evacuation
- Distance >2 hours or >200 kn from receiving hospital
- Require a medical escort

Royal Flying Doctors Service

The RFDS provides access to primary healthcare and aeromedical services across the state. They operate 24 hours a day 7 days a week. In addition to providing aeromedical retrievals of critically ill or injured patients, the RFDS also delivers a broad range of essential primary and preventative healthcare services.

Retrieval Preparation

A number of important tasks should be performed whilst awaiting aeromedical retrieval.

Ensure documentation is ready to go with the patient, this should include:

- Pre-hospital documentation
- Referral letter
- Copies of nursing/medical records
- Pathology results
- Recent sets of clinical observations
- Imaging
- If digital radiology available electronically transfer images to receiving facility

It is not always possible or practical to hand over a patient at a hospital, and it is important to determine and agree upon a location for handover as part of the retrieval co-ordination process. If the patient has been stabilised and prepared, it may be possible to perform handover at the airport/airstrip. Critically unwell and unstable patients are usually reviewed at the referring facility by the retrieval team prior to transport, and their input and expertise may be required to ensure patients are safe for transfer.

If there is room, an escort may accompany the patient at the discretion of the pilot. This is often the case when transporting children.

The following general preparations should also take place whilst awaiting transport services:

- Patient identification (apply ID bands where available).
- Record weight, height and widest point (generally not a problem in paediatric patients).
- Analgesia should be given as movement may exacerbate pain.
- An antiemetic should be considered as vomiting may exacerbate the clinical condition.
- IV access should be secured as it may be more difficult during flight due to space restrictions and turbulence.
- Consider the need for an indwelling catheter.
- Prepare required infusions e.g. fluids, antibiotics.
- Ensure NGT placed in ventilated patients or patients with bowel obstruction.

A number of specific medical conditions require special preparation, these include:

- Mental illness/disturbed behaviour, these patients may require sedation and/or physical restraint. Fortunately, this is uncommon in children.
- Infectious conditions including COVID risk should be considered prior to transfer as there is limited ability to isolate patients in small aircraft. Appropriate PPE should be worn.
- Patients with possible spinal injury may require transport on a vacuum mattress.
- Patients with possible bowel obstruction should have an NGT inserted and should be left on free drainage (not spigotted). Trapped gas will expand in volume at altitude, worsening pain. An adequately and draining NGT allows gastric gas to escape and reduce the risk of vomiting and aspiration during transfer.
- In patients with pneumothorax, an intercostal catheter should be placed and connect to a Heimlich valve or a Portex ambulatory system as trapped gas in the pleural cavity will expand at altitude resulting in respiratory compromise. It is difficult to insert an ICC during transport. Underwater seal drains are avoided due to the risk of retrograde flow during transfer.
- Patients with penetrating eye injury should be given antiemetics and may need to be transported at reduced cabin altitude as trapped gas within the globe will expand at altitude potentially worsening the injury. Vomiting may also exacerbate the injury by raising intraocular pressure.

AVIATION CONSIDERATIONS

Air travel comes with inherent challenges especially for patients with underlying health conditions. This is particularly challenge in small children where there is relatively less physiological reserve. Helicopters used for aeromedical retrieval often do not have pressurised cabins and therefore operate below 10,000 ft above sea level (FASL). Fixed-wing aircraft pressurise cabins between 7 and 8000 FASL. At sea level, the partial pressure of inspired oxygen is 149 mmHg, and this decreases as altitude rises. Relative hypoxia is common. Noise, temperature and vibration are unsettling for patients (particularly children) and distress can result in worsening of clinical status and make patients more difficult to assess. In addition to changes in partial pressure of gases with increasing altitude, specific knowledge of and compensation for changes in atmospheric pressure should be considered. The physical effects of expansion of gas-filled cavities such as the middle ear, lungs and sinuses, the gastrointestinal (GI) tract and potential spaces in the pleural space should be considered when planning a retrieval involving aeromedical transport. If the patient's condition requires it, it is possible to pressurise the cabin to near sea level; however, this prevents aircraft from reaching their cruising altitudes resulting in increased transport time and this must be balanced against the risks of physiological embarrassment from changes in pressure inside the cabin. The transport will need to be lower and slower, which reduces flying range and may expose them to increased turbulence and increased risk from adverse weather conditions.

Two main types of aircraft are available for aeromedical transfer. Helicopters are able to access more referral sites than fixed-wing aircraft but have a shorter range, and a more confined working area. They are also noisy and more prone to turbulence. Their ability to land closer to hospitals often offsets their speed differential with a fixed-wing aircraft but they are very expensive to maintain. Fixed-wing aircraft have a much greater range and are often the only option for patients located very distant from the receiving hospital. We utilise a combination of helicopter, road and fixed-wing transfers into our tertiary level hospital.

Pre-Flight Preparation

A structured assessment of airway, breathing and circulation as well as neurology and other factors is conducted prior to patient movement. There is much debate in retrieval medicine as to whether a 'scoop and run' vs a 'stay and play' approach is the best approach. Generally, an individualised approach focussed on the risks of delay vs the risk of in-flight deterioration needs to be weighed against each other.

The following factors should be considered in preparing for transfer:

- Appropriate equipment and monitoring for transfer.
- Adequate pain relief during transfer.
- A plan for in-flight deterioration should be made.
- A plan should be made for equipment failure e.g. back-up power supply.
- IV access and invasive monitoring should be secured prior to movement.

One of the most dangerous periods in the transfer is movement from the hospital into and out of the aircraft and care should be taken during this critical time period (Figure 3.2).

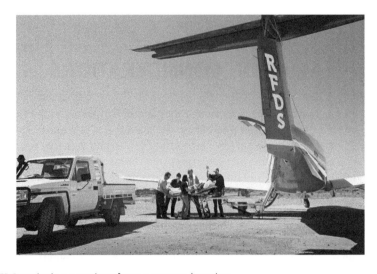

FIGURE 3.2   RFDS retrieving a patient from a remote location.

In-Flight Risks

It is necessary to conduct ongoing reassessment of the patient during transportation. Continuous direct observation is supplemented by monitored data. All personnel and the patient need to be restrained and equipment stowed during critical phases of flight, limiting rapid access. Communication is often hampered by aircraft noise. Commencement of cardiopulmonary resuscitation is very difficult and pre-emptive performance of procedures for expected deterioration such as intubation and a plan for deterioration is a vital step in reducing this risk.

Post-Flight Management

A plan needs to be made for safely offloading the patient and transfer to the definitive facility must be confirmed. The patient may need a further road transfer if arriving at an airport, which may also require a medical escort. It is obviously a key to the success of a safe transfer for all relevant team members to be kept updated as to progress of a transfer and clear and effective communication is integral to the safe transfer and retrieval of a patient.

Once the patient arrives at the destination, after introductions and identification, it is necessary to hand over to the receiving team. A structured handover is useful as it prevents missing important and valuable information.

SUMMARY

The safe and effective transport of critically unwell paediatric patients across large distances is a complex process.

The best outcomes are achieved by utilising specialists in retrieval services that have an in-depth knowledge of the available equipment, the underlying problems such as weather events and a deep understanding of the availability of specialist services in different centres. Communication between accepting and receiving teams needs to be carefully co-ordinated to ensure that patients are moved to the most appropriate centre. It is sometimes necessary for patients to undergo multiple stops in their journey, particularly when very large distances are involved. In such situations, multiple teams at multiple hospitals may need to be involved. As transport becomes more complicated, the potential for errors increases. Ultimately, careful assessment and excellent communication between senior clinicians are central in achieving the best outcomes for patients whilst reducing risks for staff and patients by preventing unnecessary or poorly co-ordinated transfers.

FURTHER READING

Johnson D, Lescombe M. Aeromedical transfer of the critically ill patient. J Intensive Care Soc. 2011;12:307–12.

Margolis SA, Ypinazar VA. Aeromedical retrieval for critical conditions: 12 years of experience with the Royal Flying Doctor Service, Queensland, Australia. J Emerg Med. 2009;36:363–8.

Milligan JE, Jones CN, Hel, DR, Munford BJ. The principles of aeromedical retrieval of the critically ill. TRens Anesth. Crit. Care. 2011;1:22–6.

Fetal Medicine

4

Daniel Carroll and Charlotte Julia Slaney

ANTENATALLY DETECTED SURGICAL PROBLEMS

It is now becoming more common to detect problems in the fetus during pregnancy. This early detection of problems has been of particular benefit in areas like Tropical North Queensland where the distance between hospitals is large and resources are unevenly allocated. Patients with known problems that will require more extensive care than can be provided locally can be appropriately counselled and where necessary the baby can be delivered in a larger centre where all the infant's immediate needs can be met.

Normal Antenatal Care

It is important to have an understanding of when scans usually occur during pregnancy and what they are intended to demonstrate.

The following ultrasounds are common in pregnancy:

- *8–9 weeks dating scan*: Some women choose to have an early ultrasound around 8–9 weeks. This may be to confirm the due date where the last menstrual period is unknown, or for reassurance.
- *11–13 weeks first trimester screen*: An ultrasound (also known as a nuchal translucency scan) combined with a blood test (PAPP-A) is recommended for all pregnant women. This is a screening test which will calculate the estimated risk of having a baby with Down syndrome and other chromosomal abnormalities. It is also commonly used to calculate the estimated due date.
- *18–20 weeks morphology scan*: An important ultrasound to check for major (physical) abnormalities. Most parents know this scan as 'the one where they find out the baby's gender'.

Extra ultrasounds beyond this may be recommended for high-risk pregnancies and/or to check on the baby's growth and wellbeing.

Commonly Detected Surgical Abnormalities in Pregnancy

A number of conditions which require paediatric surgery can be detected antenatally. It falls outside the scope of this chapter to discuss in detail the diagnosis of these conditions, and although it is not an

DOI: 10.1201/9781003156659-4

exhaustive list of problems, generally the issues encountered in clinical practice fall into one of several groups:

- Antenatally detected renal tract abnormalities
- Anterior abdominal wall defects
- Cystic thoracic lesions
- Neural tube defects (NTDs)
- Cleft lip and palate
- Congenital diaphragmatic hernia (CDH)
- Intestinal dilatation
- Cystic intra-abdominal lesions
- Abnormalities of liquor volume
- Limb abnormalities

Antenatally Detected Renal Tract Abnormalities

The commonest problem encountered in paediatric surgical practice is the patient with a pregnancy complicated by antenatally detected renal tract abnormalities. Over the past decade, an improvement in the technology for ultrasound scan (USS) has resulted in an increase in the incidence of antenatally detected renal tract abnormalities. Around 1:50 pregnancies are associated with a renal tract abnormality, the majority of these are minor and will not require surgical intervention. It is important to distinguish this from patients with more complex and serious underlying conditions that may require urgent postnatal interventions. These are discussed more fully in Chapter 10, but in general more severe and bilateral renal diseases, particularly in association with oligohydramnios, are concerning features and should be discussed further. It is often possible to make a detailed interpretation of scans taken in the first trimester, sometimes renal tract abnormalities may be easiest to identify on these scans and it is my practice to go back and look at these scans when they are available when attempting to interpret early postnatal scans. The kidneys are often visualised better in early pregnancy using the acoustic window of the amniotic fluid to get good views of the developing renal tract. It is important to consider that babies with one abnormality are more likely to have some other problems, and so they should undergo careful routine checks by a paediatrician after delivery.

The following problems are more significant than simple antenatal hydronephrosis and should prompt consideration for discussion with paediatric surgery prior to delivery:

- Bilateral moderate or severe hydronephrosis
- Oligohydramnios which may result in either moulding deformities or pulmonary insufficiency
- Suspicion of bladder exstrophy (difficult to detect antenatally unless specifically waiting for the bladder to fill)
- Hydronephrosis in a solitary kidney

Male patients with unilateral severe hydroureteronephrosis may be suffering from bladder outlet obstruction from **posterior urethral valves** (**PUVs**). These patients require urgent assessment by a neonatologist following delivery and warrant urgent postnatal investigation with USS. It is important to consider that if USS of the renal tract is performed too soon after birth, then it may be falsely reassuring. There is a relative oliguria in the first 24–48 h of life and it is possible to miss or underestimate severe urinary tract obstruction in this time period. An early scan may be useful as a baseline investigation, but should be repeated after 48 h, to ensure that this is not the case. This is particularly problematic for patients who are understandably keen to be discharged but live a long way from hospital. It is useful to manage expectations by having a guided conversation around the need and timing of investigations postnatally to allow parents to understand the need for a delayed discharge and to allow families to plan appropriately for this.

Anterior Abdominal Wall Defects

There are two major classes of abdominal wall defects which are covered in more detail in Chapter 5 on neonatal surgery. In general, they can be classified as either covered or uncovered defects.

Uncovered defects are termed **gastroschisis** (see Figure 4.1 for a postnatal picture of a baby with gastroschisis) and are far more common in our patient group than that reported in other populations, with an incidence of around 1:1000. They are almost universally associated with a defect to the right of the midline, and the bowel may be either supple or matted dependent upon the response to being exposed to amniotic fluid. For simple defects, the bowel can sometimes be reduced at the bedside with simple analgesia and appropriate nursing support. When this is possible, it removes the need for general anaesthesia, but when the bowel is very matted or there are other problems with the baby, it may be necessary to perform simple reduction under anaesthesia and closure of the defect, or to place the bowel in a silo and perform a staged reduction. It is useful to adequately counsel parents, so they understand the need for surgery immediately after birth and the likelihood of a prolonged stay in hospital, often far away from home. Families often require the support of extended family and work to facilitate this and allowing them to plan is often helpful in reducing anxieties, tensions and social problems in the immediate postnatal period. It is important to consider and address social and cultural problems that may arise from a stay away from home, particularly for indigenous patients and the involvement of the indigenous liaison officers is usually beneficial.

Most patients require intravenous feeding and gradual establishment of enteral feeding and the median length of time on parenteral nutrition is around 2 weeks. Some patients, particularly with complex gastroschisis, where there may be an associated intestinal atresia, require much longer hospital stays.

Covered defects are termed **exomphalos** and are less common (they occur in approximately 1:5000 live deliveries). These can further be divided into exomphalos major and minor, dependent upon the size of the defect. Exomphalos minor is associated with a high incidence of other abnormalities (up to 50%), and although the surgery to reduce the exomphalos and close the defect is often straightforward,

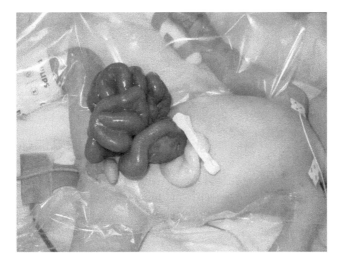

FIGURE 4.1   Neonate with gastroschisis.

the outcomes are dictated by these other abnormalities (e.g. chromosomal abnormalities, cardiac abnormalities). It is essential that babies with exomphalos minor undergo a careful postnatal examination to ensure that no other abnormalities are missed. Larger defects are more problematic surgically and may be associated with other syndromes e.g. Beckwith–Wiedemann syndrome. It is important to monitor for hypoglycaemia in the neonatal period as prolonged hypoglycaemia is associated with very poor outcomes.

In general, we would expect that patients with anterior abdominal wall defects are delivered in a centre with access to both neonatal intensive care services and paediatric surgery. The timing of delivery is important. There is known to be a significant risk of stillbirth in the latter stages of pregnancy in gastroschisis. We would recommend that patients are admitted and carefully monitored from around 36 weeks gestation and often labour is induced at around 37 weeks. Spontaneous vaginal delivery is preferable wherever possible, although a significant number of caesarean section deliveries occur.

If a patient spontaneously delivers a baby with a gastroschisis, then a number of first aid measures can be lifesaving. It is important to keep the baby '**warm**, **pink and sweet**'. Practically, this means that the bowel needs to be covered with a non-occlusive dressing (cling film is usually used), and supported so that the bowel does not become ischaemic. If the bowel will not sit in a good position with the baby supine, then it may be necessary to place the baby in a lateral position to make sure the extra-abdominal bowel loops remain well perfused. Sometimes it is easier to support the bowel with a doughnut-shaped dressing to prevent the mesenteric vessels from kinking. It is important to monitor the oxygen saturations, treat any other associated life-threatening issues and check the glucose to identify any associated hypoglycaemia. Intravenous access should be established early, and the stomach should be kept empty by passing a nasogastric tube which should be aspirated regularly.

Congenital Thoracic Malformations

A number of different conditions may present as abnormal findings within the chest on a fetal USS. The commonest of these is a congenital pulmonary airway malformation (CPAM), less commonly we may identify a bronchogenic cyst or a pulmonary sequestration. The postnatal management of these conditions is discussed elsewhere and is beyond the intended scope of this chapter.

CPAMs arise from the premature cessation of normal lung development during various stages of embryogenesis. The reported incidence of CPAM is between 1 in 10,000 and 1 in 35,000 births, although we see an incidence of around 1 in 5000 in our population in Tropical North Queensland. Most occur spontaneously and are not associated with either genetic abnormalities or problems during pregnancy. They have been classified into five major sub-types, using the Stocker classification based on their underlying pathological features (type 0–4).

Antenatally, they are typically classified on the basis of their appearance on USS and where available fetal MRI. They are divided into microcystic or macrocystic appearance. It is important to remember that although the child may not be symptomatic after birth and although the abnormality may not be visible on CXR, a follow-up CT or MRI scan should be done in the first six months of life. This should be performed urgently in children who are symptomatic. CPAM types 1 and 4 appear as one or two large air-filled cysts, type 2 appears as multiple smaller air-filled cysts. Type 3 presents as a solid homogenous mass on CXR.

It is possible to identify patients at greater risk of pulmonary insufficiency after delivery by determining the size of the CPAM in relation to the surrounding lung volume. This is termed the CPAM volume ratio. CPAM volume is estimated using the formula:

- CPAM volume = (Length × Height × Width × 0.52)

To allow for a fair value allowing for the size of the fetus to be calculated, the CPAM volume is divided by the maximal head circumference.

- A CVR ≤ 1.6 has a favourable prognosis with a low risk of developing hydrops in the absence of a dominant cyst.
- A CVR from 1.2 to 1.6 is moderate risk and is usually monitored twice weekly, a CVR <1.2 is low risk and is usually monitored weekly.
- A CVR <1.6 or one with a large dominant cyst is considered to be high risk with an increased risk of developing hydrops and is usually monitored carefully during fetal life (two to three times a week).
- A cyst is considered dominant if it is larger than one-third of the total size of the CPAM.

Fetal surgery for congenital lung lesions is controversial and not carried out in all centres. Patients with progressive fetal hydrops may benefit from interventions such as fetal surgery (usually a drainage procedure) or the antenatal administration of corticosteroids to facilitate lung maturation. In the immediate postnatal period, it may be necessary to perform emergent surgery if the child is symptomatic. Usually this is only the case when more than 20% of the hemithorax is involved. Surgery is usually considered for patients with bilateral or multifocal cysts, pneumothorax or a family history of pleuropulmonary blastoma. Often in children with minor symptoms, surgery is performed to prevent recurrent infections or for the treatment of potential malignancy in the longer term in suspected type 4 lesions. In asymptomatic patients, surgery is more controversial with some surgeons opting for a conservative approach. Either option is viable or most surgeons approach is dictated by the family's feeling towards a surgical vs a conservative approach to management.

Bronchopulmonary sequestrations

The commonest antenatally detected thoracic malformation that masquerades as a CPAM is a bronchopulmonary sequestration, they account for only around 1:20 if congenital lung malformations. These congenital malformations can appear similar to a CPAM, but there is no connection between the lesion and the tracheobronchial tree. They can arise either inside the lung tissue or outside and can occur above or below the diaphragm. They are often difficult to discriminate from a CPAM on USS unless a large feeding vessel can be seen as they receive their anomalous vascular supply from the systemic circulation in the case of extra-lobar sequestrations. Antenatal or postnatal cross-sectional imaging is usually helpful in discriminating between these lesions. Approximately two-thirds of all these lesions occur in the left lower lobe. In a fetus with progressive hydrops, thoraco-amniotic shunting may be considered. Following delivery, it is possible for babies with large volume sequestrations to demonstrate significant respiratory compromise and the use of high-frequency oscillatory ventilation (HFOV) or extracorporeal membrane oxygenation (ECMO) may be necessary. In such cases, early surgical resection is usually performed once stabilisation is achieved. Poor prognostic factors include:

- Fetal hydrops
- Pulmonary hypoplasia
- Large pleural effusions

Patients with extra-lobar intra-abdominal sequestrations have a better prognosis although it is important to consider the differential diagnosis of neuroblastoma.

Bronchogenic cysts

These are rare lesions with a prevalence of around 1:50,000 live births, they are classified dependent upon their location, they are most commonly mediastinal or intrapulmonary, and mediastinal cysts are further classified into:

- Paratracheal
- Paraoesophageal
- Carinal
- Hilar
- Miscellaneous locations

More rarely, they can occur in the pleura, neck, diaphragm, retroperitoneum or pericardium. Treatment depends upon the location of the cyst and whether there are symptoms. Most surgeons recommend complete resection to prevent complications.

Summary

The outcome for antenatally detected thoracic abnormalities is usually excellent. It is important whenever possible to allow the family to meet with and discuss postnatal management strategies with paediatric surgeons prior to delivery. In a large geographical area like ours, it is possible to facilitate these conversations via telehealth to avoid unnecessary disruptions to the family. In general, a multidisciplinary approach to helping the family is useful, and where necessary conversations with neonatologists, indigenous liaison officers, local paediatricians and social workers can be helpful to determine the resources that will be needed to achieve the best outcomes for the family.

Spina Bifida

Spina bifida is a type of **neural tube defect** (NTD) where the baby's spine and spinal cord does not develop normally during fetal life. There are three main types of spina bifida: myelomeningocele (MMC), lipomeningocele and spina bifida occulta. Spina bifida is often diagnosed antenatally. They are important to the paediatric surgeon and paediatric urologist as there is often a significant degree of bladder and bowel dysfunction requiring surgery and conservative strategies to be implemented to provide for the best long-term outcomes for patients. Many cases are identified during routine antenatal care either as a result of an abnormal prenatal sonogram or because of an elevated maternal alpha-fetoprotein. It is important to consider the potential for spina bifida in patients with risk factors for neural tube defects. These include:

- Having a sibling with spina bifida
- Having a mother with spina bifida
- Deficit folic acid in the maternal diet before pregnancy
- Exposure to certain medications in pregnancy (e.g. sodium valproate)

Spina bifida in Australia is less common since the introduction of mandatory folic acid fortification of wheat flour on 13 September 2009. NTDs are reported in around 1:5000 live births in Australia with around 150 new patients born every year. These patients are not evenly distributed across Australia and are far more common in disadvantaged groups with poorer health literacy and poorer access to healthcare resources.

Myelomeningocele

This is the commonest neural tube defect. Neural tube closure occurs early in pregnancy, and problems resulting in MMC are thought to date from around the third week of fetal life. A child with MMC presents with a fluid-filled sac attached to the back. There is most often a defect in the skin as well. The bones of the spine fail to develop and do not close around the spinal cord, the sac protrudes through this defect exposing the delicate spinal roots. Children born with MMC have associated muscle weakness and decreased sensation, with higher lesions resulting in worse outcomes.

Lipomeningocele

This type of spina bifida is associated with an overlying fatty tumour. At birth, the skin is intact overlying the spinal cord and vertebral anomaly. The lower the level of the spinal cord defect the better the long-term prognosis.

Spina bifida occulta

Typically, this is an incidental finding. The lowest lumbar vertebrae are found to have a small midline defect. There are often no long-term consequences from this condition, and this is often incidentally diagnosed. There is an association with anorectal malformations, it is not typically diagnosed antenatally.

Postnatal treatment and evaluation

In cases of open MMC, the neural tube defect is closed in the first 48 h of life by a neurosurgeon. Many specialists are involved in the care of a child with spina bifida, and it often involves a long-term relationship particularly with paediatric surgeons and urologists. A multidisciplinary approach is preferred with neurosurgery, orthopaedics, paediatric urology and surgery, physiotherapists, paediatricians and neonatologists. Once the child has recovered from emergent neurosurgery, it is important to protect the detrusor and help achieve optimal bladder and bowel outcomes for the child in the longer term. Practically, this usually involves the early institution of clean intermittent catheterisation to protect the bladder and kidneys from early long-term damage. This is often difficult for families, and antenatal counselling of families by surgical teams to explain the value of such treatment is often enormously helpful in allowing families to prepare.

Fetal surgery for neural tube defects

Fetal surgery for spina bifida has shown enormous promise. The early results from surgery are most encouraging although it is offered at only a few larger centres currently. There are significant risks to the fetus from such surgery as well as risks to the mother, but in the future, it may become more commonplace.

Cleft Lip and Palate

Abnormalities of the facial cleft are relatively common, with around 1 in 700 live births having an abnormality of either the lip or palate. It is more common in males than females. In around 50% of cases, both the lip and palate are affected, in 25% only the lip and in 25% only the palate. It is unilateral in around 75% of cases and bilateral in around 25%.

The typical cleft lip appears as a linear defect extending from one side of the lip into the nostril. It is often visible on the first USS at 11–13 weeks. In a cleft palate, there is an extension of this defect through the alveolar ridge and hard palate, reaching the floor of the nasal cavity or even the floor of the orbit. Diagnosis of isolated cleft palate is more difficult. Targeted examination of the retronasal triangle in a coronal view and the maxillary gap in the standard mid-sagittal view of the face can allow for identification during routine screening.

Chromosomal abnormalities (most commonly trisomies 13 and 18) are found in around 1–2% of cases. Unilateral cleft lip is not associated with chromosomal abnormalities. Facial cleft abnormalities have a strong association with a large number of syndromes. Around 30% of total cases are associated with another syndrome. The most common are **Treacher Collins syndrome**, **Goldenhar syndrome** or **Pierre Robin sequence**.

Because of these associated problems, it is recommended that patients in whom facial cleft abnormalities are detected antenatally undergo detailed USS examination and invasive testing for karyotyping and array.

Although there is no necessity for anything other than standard obstetric care and delivery, it is likely that the baby will have feeding difficulties and consideration should be given to delivery in a tertiary-level centre. In patients with more complex facial cleft abnormalities, the need for surgery and the treatment by a multidisciplinary team for associated problems in the longer term mean that there is often value in seeing a paediatric surgeon for antenatal counselling for the family to discuss the role and timing of surgery postnatally.

Surgical repair is usually commenced at around 3–6 months of age, and for patients with a cleft lip, it is important to strap the edges of the lip together to improve the ability to feed and also to improve the size of the defect. The benefit of being in a tertiary-level centre at this stage of the management is clear, and also helps the family to meet members of the surgical team to discuss timing and nature of further surgeries.

Congenital Diaphragmatic Hernia

CDH occurs when the diaphragm fails to develop normally during fetal life. The diaphragm normally forms at between the 7th and 10th week of gestation. This condition is discussed in much greater detail elsewhere in this book, but briefly we will describe the features seen during pregnancy and the management in the antenatal period.

CDH occurs in approximately 1 in 3000–5000 live births. There is a slight female preponderance and familial clusters have been seen but are uncommon. The risk of further pregnancies being affected is around 1:50, unless CDH is seen as part of a syndrome. There are several different forms of diaphragmatic hernia; the most common type is a Bochdalek hernia which accounts for around 90% of all cases. These are usually on the left side. Morgagni hernias are less common and are found behind the sternum. In some patients, the diaphragm may remain intact but has an attenuated portion resulting in an eventration.

More than half of patients are able to be diagnosed antenatally. In addition to confirmation of diagnosis, it is important that pregnancies complicated by this condition are offered further expert assessment of the condition and provided with suitable information to guide decisions during pregnancy. Associated anomalies occur in around 50% of all pregnancies; these include cardiac defects (52%), genitourinary abnormalities (23%), gastrointestinal abnormalities (14%) and central nervous system (CNS) anomalies (10%).

It is useful to consider which patients are likely to have good outcomes. The following factors are linked to a positive prognosis:

- Left-sided diaphragmatic hernia
- No other associated anomalies
- A larger observed/expected lung-to-head ratio (LHR) (>45%)

Because we know that these features are associated with positive outcomes, antenatal management is guided by trying to identify those who are more at risk immediately after birth. At the initial appointment with the fetal medicine team, the side of the defect, liver and stomach position are assessed. The woman will be counselled regarding CDH and will be offered karyotyping. Options for management of pregnancy are discussed and are often guided by the results of scan findings and the presence of associated anomalies.

In order to evaluate fetal lung volume, LHR is calculated. This is obtained by measuring the size of the contralateral lung and considering it in proportion to the head circumference – this can be calculated by either measure in the longest axis or the AP diameter. The degree of lung hypoplasia correlates well with the observed/expected LHR.

Ultrasonography is the major imaging modality used in the assessment of CDH; however, fetal MRI may have a role in providing additional information to aid parental decision-making.

In selected patients with normal karyotype fetal intervention by occluding the trachea to accelerate, lung growth can be considered. This is currently not offered in our centre. Occlusion of the trachea causes entrapment of lung fluid resulting in increased pressure in the developing lung. Early clinical trials have demonstrated some success in neonatal survival at the expense of a higher incidence of preterm labour and premature rupture of membranes (PROM) and preterm delivery.

Patients with known CDH prior to birth should be considered for management with steroids from around 34th week of gestation to improve lung maturation. Delivery should be planned for around 39th week of gestation in a tertiary centre with paediatric surgery and NICU availability. Postnatal management of CDH is discussed in more detail in Chapter 5 on neonatal surgical conditions.

Summary

- CDH is a rare condition present in around 1:5000 live births.
- There is a high risk of associated anomalies being present.
- Delivery should be in a tertiary centre and families should be moved to a tertiary centre prior to delivery.
- Maternal steroid administration should be considered from 34 weeks' gestation.

Intestinal Dilatation

Another common antenatal abnormality is the unexplained presence of dilated loops bowel antenatally. A number of different causes must be considered but often there is a transient dilatation of one or several loops of bowel seen on a scan that subsequently resolves. As long as there are no other abnormalities these patients require no specific interventions postnatally.

A small number of patients have a persistent or progressive dilatation of intestinal loops antenatally. For those with only a single dilated loop with a large gastric bubble in the right upper quadrant, we must consider the possibility of duodenal atresia (see Figure 4.2). This should in turn lead us to look carefully for features of trisomy 21 because of the frequent association of duodenal atresia with T21.

Another potential cause of progressive bowel dilatation is a partially obstructed bowel loop due to an intestinal duplication cyst. When the lumen of the bowel is completely interrupted as in intestinal atresia, we may expect to see dilated loops of proximal bowel, although frequently in intestinal atresia there are no abnormal findings seen on the routine antenatal images in the first and second trimesters.

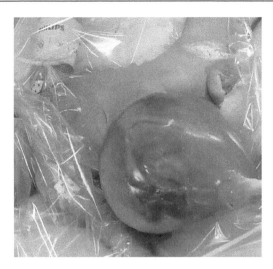

FIGURE 4.2   Neonate with exomphalos.

Cystic intra-abdominal lesions

Sometimes it is possible to demonstrate a cystic structure in the abdominal cavity on antenatal scans. These may resolve spontaneously as pregnancy progresses, but they may be persistent and progressive and in such cases, further investigation is warranted postnatally. The commonest causes of intra-abdominal cystic lesions are:

- Intestinal duplications
- Rare neonatal tumours e.g. germ cell tumours, teratoma, neuroblastoma, sacro-coccygeal tumours (SCT)
- Ovarian cystic disease in females

The size and exact nature of the cystic lesion after birth is important in dictating the need for further investigations. In general, larger (>5 cm diameter) and complex cystic lesion of the ovary require urgent removal because of the risk of adnexal torsion or underlying malignancy. The management of potential neonatal tumours is discussed in more detail elsewhere in the book.

Abnormalities in amniotic fluid volume

Oligohydramnios is defined as a decreased amniotic fluid volume (AFV) relative to gestational age. Conversely polyhydramnios is an increase in AFV. AFV is calculated by one of two methods, the amniotic fluid index (AFI) or the maximum vertical pocket (MVP). The MVP tends to overdiagnose polyhydramnios and AFI tends to underdiagnose oligohydramnios.

The volume of amniotic fluid in the gestational sac is a result of a balance between fluid movement out of the sac and fluid production. In the first half of pregnancy, lung secretions and osmotic and hydrostatic transport of maternal plasma across fetal membranes account for the majority of amniotic fluid production. From around 16th week of gestation, the fetal kidneys begin to produce fluid becoming the major contributor towards amniotic fluid production towards the end of pregnancy.

Abnormalities in AFV are found in around 5% of all pregnancies, with oligohydramnios present in around 4% and polyhydramnios present in around 1%. It is important to investigate patients with AFV abnormalities as these may be an important signal of problems with pregnancy that need to be managed antenatally.

Differential diagnoses

Oligohydramnios

- Idiopathic/unexplained (50%)
- Placental causes
  - Abruption, twin–twin transfusion syndrome
- Maternal causes
  - Uteroplacental insufficiency
  - Hypertension
  - Thrombophilia
  - Preeclampsia
- Drugs
  - ACE inhibitors
  - NSAIDs
  - Cocaine use
- Fetal causes
  - Premature preterm rupture of membranes (1:3 of cases)
  - Renal tract abnormalities (obstructive nephropathy, PUV)
  - Post-term pregnancies
  - Chromosomal abnormalities

As a paediatric surgeon, it is most likely that we will be consulted in patients with demonstrable surgical causes of oligohydramnios such as genitourinary abnormalities. In patients with antenatal hydronephrosis and oligohydramnios, obstructive uropathy should be considered and appropriate steps taken to plan for initial management postnatally. This is discussed in more detail in Chapter 10 on paediatric urology.

Polyhydramnios
There are a large number of unrelated conditions that can result in polyhydramnios. The most common causes are:

- Fetal causes
  - Fetal malformations e.g. TOF/OA, CDH
  - Genetic disease, including chromosomal abnormalities
  - Fetal anaemia
  - Fetal infections (e.g. parvovirus B19, rubella, CMV, syphilis)
  - Neuromuscular disorders
- Maternal causes
  - Gestational diabetes mellitus (GDM)
  - Multiple pregnancies

Management of Amniotic Fluid Volume Abnormalities

Idiopathic and mild abnormalities of AFV are common and require no specific intervention. Generally, these are picked up incidentally later in pregnancy and are mild.

More extreme variations in liquor volume are more likely to be due to an underlying problem with either the fetus or some complication of pregnancy. It is recommended for patients with severe oligohydramnios or polyhydramnios that delivery occurs in a tertiary-level facility due to the potential for maternal and neonatal morbidity and mortality. The consultation with a maternal-fetal medicine specialist is indicated for patients with severe polyhydramnios for assessment for reductive amniocentesis and treatment of twin–twin transfusion syndrome.

Patients with significant oligohydramnios are at increased risk of secondary pulmonary hypoplasia (Potter's syndrome) as well as club foot and other moulding deformities. It is important to ensure that wherever possible these patients are delivered at a centre capable of providing high-level neonatal support.

OVERVIEW OF CURRENT MANAGEMENT OF ANTENATALLY DETECTED SURGICAL PROBLEMS

Advances in ultrasonography have led to an increased rate of detection of surgical problems antenatally. One abnormal finding should prompt more detailed and often more frequent scanning as further unidentified problems are more likely. The involvement of maternal-fetal medicine consultants is useful in identifying problems and appropriately involving other teams that will be involved in care postnatally. This allows families to make informed decisions surrounding management in pregnancy and allows them to gather information prior to delivery about the likely outcomes.

Antenatal counselling requires an in-depth knowledge of the natural history of these conditions and their likely management. It is almost always helpful for families to meet members of the paediatric surgical team prior to delivery. Early identification of problems allows local teams to be involved at an early stage and facilitates communication between departments.

FURTHER READING

Davenport M, Coppi PD, editors. Chapter 3: Fetal medicine and surgery. In Paediatric Surgery. 2nd Edition. 73–102. Oxford University Press; 2021.

Lakhoo K. Fetal counselling for surgical congenital malformations. In: Puri P, Hollwarth M, editors. Paediatric Surgery. Springer; 2009.

The Neonatal Surgical Patient

5

Kiera Roberts, Harry Stalewski and Daniel Carroll

INTRODUCTION

The complexity of embryological and fetal development may lead to a wide range of congenital anomalies requiring surgical correction early in life. These conditions may be seen in isolation, or often in conjunction with other conditions as part of a syndrome, sequence or association (such as the VACTERL association, including vertebral, anorectal, cardiac, tracheo-(o)esophageal, renal and limb anomalies).

Neonatal surgical conditions in some cases may be diagnosed or suspected antenatally and require immediate postnatal management and intervention. Many conditions, however, may not be evident on antenatal imaging and may only present after birth, necessitating a thorough knowledge of the normal anatomy and physiology of the newborn, and the significance of deviations from this normal course (such as delayed passage of meconium in the diagnosis of Hirschsprung disease).

In general, neonatal surgical patients present in one of three following ways:

- Antenatal-diagnosed abnormalities
- After investigation for other abnormalities picked up after birth
- Signs of acute surgical problems, e.g. abdominal distension, bile-stained vomiting, blood PR

Of these, the most important is **bile-stained vomiting**. Any neonate with bile-stained vomiting should be considered to have an acute surgical pathology until proven otherwise and requires prompt referral and appropriate assessment to rule out a surgical pathology.

For our patient population, it is important to identify patients with potential paediatric surgical problems prior to delivery wherever possible. Improvements in antenatal scanning have resulted in more patients being identified with congenital anomalies than ever before. The presence of one abnormality should prompt further detailed scans as the identification of further abnormalities make the presence of surgical problems much more likely. It is often safer to transfer patients with known surgical problems prior to delivery as neonatal transport can be difficult and the early availability of neonatal intensive care and paediatric surgery has been shown to improve outcomes.

The increasing effectiveness of neonatal care for very small babies has led to an increased incidence of problems related to prematurity. In particular, we see far more inguinal hernias in premature babies as well as the ever-present risk of necrotising enterocolitis (NEC).

DOI: 10.1201/9781003156659-5

GENERAL CONSIDERATIONS

Surgical conditions that affect the newborn pose unique challenges in management due to the physiology of the neonate. The extremely premature neonate, for example, may be both at greater risk of developing surgical conditions due to their immature physiology (such as NEC), as well as adding complexity to the management of other congenital conditions.

In terms of neonatal physiology, within the first moments of extra-uterine life, the newborn begins the transition from fetal to neonatal circulation, with the first breaths resulting in transition from placental to pulmonary gas exchange, a significant decrease in the pulmonary vascular resistance and increase in the systemic vascular resistance due to removal of the placenta from circulation. Fetal circulation is marked by three structures allowing shunting of blood: the *foramen ovale* between the right and left atrium, the ductus arteriosus between the left pulmonary artery and aorta, and the ductus venosus between the left umbilical vein and inferior vena cava. Postnatally, these shunts typically close rapidly; however, persistence of the fetal circulation may be seen in conditions such as congenital diaphragmatic hernia (CDH) with its associated pulmonary hypertension.

Pulmonary development continues after birth well into childhood, and the immature respiratory system of the newborn may pose challenges to ventilatory management during general anaesthetic and in the neonatal intensive care unit. Renal function also continues to develop postnatally, with the concentrating capacity of both preterm and full-term neonates being well below that of adults.

Newborns, particularly premature neonates, have difficulty maintaining their body temperature, due in part, to their relatively large surface area, poor thermal regulation and small body mass. This may be of particular significance in conditions such as gastroschisis with exposure of the bowel, as well as with exposure of the neonate during any surgical procedure necessitating a warmed theatre.

Neonates with surgical pathologies are at high risk for hypoglycaemia, in addition to those who are premature, small for gestational age, or born to mothers with maternal gestational diabetes. Signs of hypoglycaemia can be subtle and difficult to detect but, in the most severe cases, may lead to seizures and coma. Careful monitoring and provision of glucose is therefore vital, particularly in the fasting patient.

NEONATAL SURGICAL CONDITIONS: A SUMMARY

Oesophageal Atresia and Tracheo-Oesophageal Fistula

Oesophageal atresia (OA), with or without tracheo-oesophageal fistula (TOF), represents the most common congenital anomaly affecting the oesophagus with a reported incidence of around 1 in 4000 live births. Following five types are described in the Gross classification:

- Type A describes an isolated esphageal atresia without fistula, accounting for approximately 10% of cases
- Type B describes oesophageal atresia with a proximal fistula
- Type C (accounting for 85% of cases) describes oesophageal atresia with a distal fistula
- Type D (oesophageal atresia with proximal and distal fistulas)
- Type E anomalies (isolated tracheo-oesophageal fistula)

Types D and E are very uncommon.

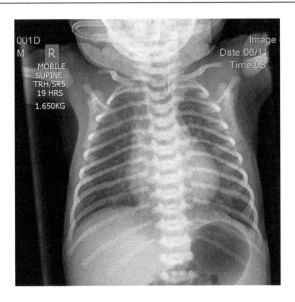

FIGURE 5.1   Chest radiograph of neonate with OA/TOF.

Antenatally, suspicion for OA/TOF may be raised with evidence of a small stomach or presence of polyhydramnios, along with other features of the VACTERL association such as cardiac defects. Most cases, however, are not evident until after birth, where the infant will be unable to feed or swallow their secretions, this is classically described as frothy secretions at the lips. Attempted passage of a naso- or oro-gastric tube will lead to coiling within the upper pouch which will be evident on a chest radiograph (see Figure 5.1). Presence of distal gas within the abdomen on X-ray is indicative of a distal fistula, whereas a gasless abdomen may be consistent with isolated oesophageal atresia and potential concern for a long gap.

In the stable infant, surgical intervention can be approached in a planned manner following further work-up with echocardiogram, as well as screening for other features of VACTERL postoperatively. Some infants, however, may be unable to be stabilised due to passage of air down the fistula resulting in progressive gastric distension and respiratory compromise, particularly premature infants. Continuous positive pressure ventilation should be avoided in these infants for this reason. In the unstable neonate, emergent thoracotomy and ligation of the fistula may be required in order to achieve stability.

Approach to the surgical repair of oesophageal atresia may be either via a right thoracotomy, or thoracoscopically, dependent on the size of the baby and surgeon preference. This approach may vary in the scenario of a right-sided aortic arch identified preoperatively, where some surgeons would approach from the left, whereas others would maintain a right-sided approach.

The procedure involves identification and ligation of the tracheo-oesophageal fistula and formation of an oesophageal anastomosis. The management of long gap oesophageal atresia is more difficult. Little consensus exists as to the exact definition of 'long gap', which is variably described by vertebral body length or centimetre measurement; however, it essentially represents the group of infants where a primary repair is not possible. Various management strategies have evolved to deal with this difficult scenario. Formation of a gastrostomy and performance of a delayed primary anastomosis after allowing a period of oesophageal lengthening is well described. Active lengthening techniques such as the use of internal or external fixation traction sutures, such as the Foker technique, have also been increasingly performed and may shorten the period of time until anastomosis can be performed. Where these techniques are unsuccessful, oesophageal replacement techniques such as gastric tube, gastric transposition or intestinal interposition may be required.

Postoperatively, anastomotic leak and stricture formation are among the most common complications with some infants requiring serial dilatations for management of the anastamotic strictures. In the longer term, these children may commonly experience symptoms such as dysphagia as well as the complications of gastro-oesophageal reflux disease and chronic respiratory infections.

In general, it is useful for a non-specialist to have a basic understanding and approach to a patient with suspected oesophageal atresia. After failed passage of an oral tube in a baby that seems unable to swallow secretions, the following steps should be performed:

- Call for senior help and ensure that IV access is established and that the baby is appropriately resuscitated, and the airway is secure.
- Order a portable chest and abdominal radiograph to determine the position of the OGT and also to look for the presence of gas below the diaphragm, where it is absent there is the possibility of long gap oesophageal atresia.
- Once the diagnosis is confirmed, then paediatric surgical services should be contacted for further advice and input into management, including organisation of a safe transfer.
- A Replogle tube may be useful in allowing drainage of the upper pouch and preventing or reducing the risk of spillover of unswallowed secretions from the upper pouch into the airway.
- Ventilation should be avoided wherever possible as positive pressure ventilation can result in progressive rapid abdominal distension and respiratory compromise.
- A careful check should be made for other anomalies, including cardiac and anorectal anomalies.

The long-term outcomes for patients with oesophageal atresia are excellent; however, it is important to consider the long-term complications of stricture development, ongoing gastro-oesophageal reflux and difficulty in swallowing. It is routine in our practice for patients to undergo a contrast swallow following surgery prior to initiation of feeds to exclude a leak at the site of the oesophageal anastamosis. Patients are also commenced on proton-pump inhibitors after surgery and continue on these medicines after discharge.

Congenital Diaphragmatic Hernia

CDH occurs due to incomplete development of the diaphragm, resulting in a defect that allows herniation of the abdominal contents into the thoracic cavity. Globally, the incidence is approximately 2.3 per 10,000 live births. The defect is typically posterolateral (Bochdalek hernia), with anterior defects (Morgagni hernia) occurring uncommonly and with a potential association with other ventral body wall defects (Pentalogy of Cantrell). CDH is associated with pulmonary hypoplasia and pulmonary hypertension and it is these pathologies that confer the mortality and morbidity of the condition. Previously theorised to develop solely due to mechanical compression from the herniated abdominal contents, increasing evidence suggests that there is also early embryonic maldevelopment of the pulmonary vasculature and parenchyma prior to diaphragmatic development (dual-hit hypothesis). Other associated anomalies may be seen, most commonly cardiac defects with major cardiac lesions portending a worse prognosis. Anomalies of the urogenital, musculoskeletal and neurological systems are also commonly encountered, as well as potential chromosomal anomalies.

CDH may be diagnosed antenatally in most cases and requires ongoing counselling and monitoring throughout gestation. In terms of prognostication, the observed to expected lung-to-head ratio (O/E LHR) provides an estimate of severity, with an O/E LHR of less than 25% being considered severe. Fetal MRI with calculation of total fetal lung volume may also be utilised. Fetal intervention (fetoscopic endoluminal tracheal occlusion) to stimulate lung growth has been demonstrated to improve survival in the severe group for those with isolated, left-sided CDH and may be of benefit in limited and select cases. It is important wherever possible that patients with suspected CDH are delivered in a centre where paediatric surgery is available as postnatal transfer of these patients can be very difficult.

Postnatally, management of infants with CDH involves careful stabilisation and ventilation, balancing the goal of appropriate oxygenation and ventilation with the risk of barotrauma to the developing neonatal lungs. Various gentle ventilation strategies are therefore utilised including high-frequency oscillatory ventilation, with a moderate degree of hypercarbia accepted in order to minimise barotrauma.

Adjunct medical therapies such as the use of sildenafil or the use of nitric oxide can be used in the management of pulmonary hypertension. Extracorporeal membrane oxygenation (ECMO) may be utilised in infants who cannot be stabilised. The role of ECMO in this cohort remains controversial, however, without clear evidence to demonstrate a survival benefit in infants with CDH. The timing of surgery in an infant on ECMO is also controversial, with some authors advocating an early repair prior to the onset of oedema, others advocating late repair on ECMO just prior to decannulation to allow for the period of peri-operative instability, and others preferring delaying surgical intervention until after decannulation.

In general, surgical repair is ideally delayed until the infant has demonstrated a period of physiological stability. Surgical repair of the defect may then be undertaken via an abdominal or thoracoscopic approach; however, minimally invasive approaches have been demonstrated to be associated with higher recurrence rates. The goal of the procedure is safe reduction of the abdominal contents from the chest, and repair of the diaphragm either primarily or using a substitute patch or muscle flap in larger defects. There is little evidence to support the use of any one patch type over another.

Long-term outcomes of surviving children are variable. Issues such as respiratory complications, gastro-oesophageal reflux disease and neurodevelopmental delay are common, and these children should have ongoing follow-up and review. It is most usual for them to be reviewed by a respiratory paediatrician on an ongoing basis after discharge as they often demonstrate significant airway irritability with significant reversible airflow limitation particularly when very young in the context of simple viral illnesses. Longer-term assessment of respiratory physiology and appropriate medical management are useful.

After an antenatal diagnosis of suspected CDH is made by the fetal medicine team, the following steps are important in management:

- Discussion between fetal medicine/paediatric surgery to stratify risk and discuss options.
- Antenatal counselling with paediatric surgery/neonatal team is offered.
- A plan is made for delivery in a centre with available paediatric surgery.
- Once the baby is born, they are assessed and resuscitated by the neonatal team.
- IV access is established and maintained.
- An NGT/OGT is passed, and the stomach kept empty to prevent gaseous distension.
- Postnatal investigations include detailed cardiac assessment and careful examination for other anomalies.
- Once the baby has demonstrated physiological stability, a plan is made for surgical repair.

Congenital Lung Lesions

Congenital lung lesions represent a spectrum of disease, including congenital pulmonary airway malformations (CPAMs), bronchopulmonary sequestrations (BPS), hybrid lesions, congenital lobar emphysema (CLE) and bronchogenic cysts. These conditions are discussed in more detail in Chapter 11 on paediatric thoracic surgery in this book.

CPAMs represent the most commonly identified antenatal lung masses and are characterised by an abnormal proliferation of the terminal respiratory structures, typically seen in the lower lobes. Antenatally these lesions may be classified as either microcystic (cysts less than 5 mm in diameter) or macrocystic (single or multiple cysts greater than 5 mm). Following detection on antenatal imaging, regression may be seen on serial ultrasound during the second and third trimester due to relative growth of the fetus in relation to the lung mass. Some lesions, however, may increase in size substantially resulting in compression of thoracic and mediastinal structures and potential development of hydrops – a condition in which large amounts of fluid build up in tissues and organs causing extensive oedema. Fetal intervention may be required in these uncommon scenarios and includes steroid administration for microcystic lesions or thoraco-amniotic shunting for macrocystic lesions. Postnatally, CPAMs may be classified by their location of development according to the Stocker classification, including type 0 (tracheobronchial), type 1 (bronchial/bronchiolar, representing the majority of cases), type 2 (bronchiolar), type 3 (bronchiolar/alveolar) and type 4 (distal acinar).

A small percentage of infants may be symptomatic secondary to the CPAM at birth with features of respiratory distress requiring early surgical intervention. Management of the asymptomatic patient is more controversial, with some authors advocating for resection of all lesions due to the potential risk of complications such as infection as well as concern for future malignancy, although this risk is, however, not clearly defined. Other authors suggest a more selective approach with resection limited to large lesions causing compressive effects or following episodes of infection. Differentiation of a simple CPAM from pleuropulmonary blastoma must also be considered, with a particular relationship noted with type 4 CPAMs (large, multi-loculated cystic lesions).

BPS, similar to CPAMs, also represent an abnormal proliferation of pulmonary tissue. Unlike CPAMs, however, they are not connected to the airway, and their vascular supply arises from the systemic rather than the pulmonary circulation. These lesions can be divided into intra-lobar (invested within the pleura of the adjacent lung and with pulmonary venous drainage) or extra-lobar lesions, which drain via systemic veins and are invested completely within their own pleural lining and may be found outside the thoracic cavity, including within or below the diaphragm. Given these, lesions do not connect with the airway, infection is seen less commonly than with CPAMs.

Hybrid lesions may, however, be seen which contain elements of both CPAMs and BPS.

CLE is uncommon and results secondary to air entrapment within a pulmonary lobe where a 'ball-valve effect' allows air to enter the lobe but not be exhaled. This leads to overdistension and permanent damage to the alveoli. The aetiology of this condition is variable, with around half thought to be idiopathic and half resulting from extrinsic compression or an intrinsic abnormality such as abnormal bronchial cartilage. CLE is rarely diagnosed antenatally, more commonly presenting after birth once the baby begins to spontaneously breathe. Mass effect from the over-distended lobe may in some cases lead to respiratory collapse requiring emergent intervention with thoracotomy and resection of the affected lobe (typically the left upper lobe). Milder forms may present later in infancy with symptoms such as recurrent respiratory infections or poor feeding.

Bronchogenic cysts are fluid or mucus-filled lesions arising from the posterior membranous wall of the airway secondary to abnormal budding from the primitive oesophageal and tracheo-bronchial tree. These lesions may be seen antenatally and potentially may cause compressive effects if large. Postnatally, lesions may be identified following episodes of infection, or obstruction of the airway or oesophagus with increasing size. Malignancy within the cyst (typically adenocarcinoma) has also been reported, albeit rarely. Surgical excision is recommended for these lesions with approach depending on the location (mediastinal or intra-parenchymal).

In general, it is uncommon for antenatally diagnosed congenital lung lesions to require emergency surgery in the neonatal period. The exceptions are the small number of cases where there is a large lesion resulting in respiratory compromise. The following steps are recommended following antenatal diagnosis of a congenital lung lesion:

- A discussion between the fetal medicine and neonatal/paediatric surgery teams to make a clear plan for delivery and immediate postnatal management.
- The family are offered antenatal counselling to discuss potential diagnoses and management.
- Following delivery in a centre offering paediatric surgery, the patient is assessed by the neonatal team.
- A chest radiograph/ultrasound scan (USS) is performed early but it is important to remember that this will not always show even some persistent large abnormalities.
- If the child is well then plans are made for further radiology (usually CT scan) after discussion with the paediatric radiology team to define anatomy.
- The patient is followed up by the paediatric surgical team for ongoing assessment of the congenital lung lesion and consideration of surgery.

Intestinal Atresias

Atresia of the intestinal tract may be seen in the fore-, mid- and hind-gut and may be single or multiple. Aetiology and management of bowel atresias differ depending on the site, and presence of one or multiple atretic segments.

Duodenal Atresia

Duodenal atresia has traditionally been theorised to occur secondary to failure of recanalisation of the duodenum during development, although this has been challenged by more recent evidence. Three types are described: type I (mucosal atresia or windsock with an intact muscular wall), type II (complete atresia with the two sections of the duodenum connected by a fibrous cord) and type III (complete separation of the duodenum). It occurs in around 1 in 5–10,000 live births and is commonly associated with chromosomal anomalies in up to 30%, in particular, trisomy 21. Other anomalies are also frequently seen in association, including gastrointestinal (such as annular pancreas, OA/TOF, anorectal anomalies, malrotation or other intestinal atresia), cardiac, renal or vertebral anomalies.

The classical appearance of duodenal atresia on imaging is the 'double bubble', with distension of the stomach and duodenum proximal to the point of obstruction (see Figure 5.2). Antenatally, polyhydramnios is also commonly seen which may lead to premature delivery. When duodenal atresia is suspected, either antenatally or postnatally, further work-up including an echocardiogram and karyotyping should be undertaken. Postnatally the neonate may develop vomiting, which may be bilious or non-bilious depending on the relationship of the atretic segment to the opening of the common bile duct.

Management of duodenal atresia involves surgical correction, typically a duodeno-duodenostomy is performed, which may be undertaken either by either a laparoscopic or open approach. Postoperatively delayed emptying of the duodenum is commonly seen with slow progression of feeds. Long-term survival

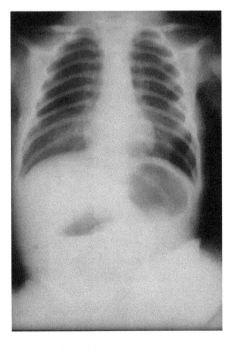

FIGURE 5.2   Radiograph of a neonate with duodenal atresia.

and quality of life is generally good, with morbidity primarily being relayed to co-morbidities. The principal immediate steps in the management of suspected duodenal atresia are outlined in the following:

- Once duodenal atresia suspected a discussion between the fetal medicine and neonatal and surgical teams take place to plan postnatal management.
- The family are offered antenatal counselling with paediatric surgery to discuss postnatal management.
- Further investigations take place to look for chromosomal abnormalities and other anomalies.
- Following delivery at a centre where paediatric surgery is available, the patient is assessed and resuscitated by the neonatal team.
- An NGT/OGT should be placed and kept on free drainage.
- An abdominal radiograph will usually confirm the presence of a double bubble appearance and later films will confirm there is no distal gas (some patients may have small amounts of distal gas with either a windsock or a small connection between proximal and distal duodenum through the ampulla of Vater).
- A careful check should be made for other anomalies (particularly cardiac and anorectal anomalies as well as looking for other features of T21).
- Once the patient is stable and the diagnosis is confirmed, an operation to correct the duodenal atresia should be performed.
- Plans should be made for TPN and an extended period of being unable to tolerate feeds may occur (even with the placement of trans-anastomotic tube).

Small Bowel Atresia

Jejunal and ileal atresia are seen in around 1 in 5000 live births, which are thought to result from a vascular insult during development leading to ischaemia of a segment of gut and subsequent development of intestinal atresia.

Four types are described:

- Type I defects have an obstructing membrane with an intact muscular wall.
- Type II describes disruption in the bowel wall with a fibrous band connecting the two segments.
- Type III describes a complete gap in continuity with a defect in the mesentery and can be further subdivided into type IIIa (simple atresia as described) and IIIb ('apple-peel' defect where the bowel is foreshortened and coiled around its blood supply from a single vessel.
- Type IV involves the presence of multiple atresias.

Unlike duodenal atresia, other extra-intestinal anomalies are less common.

Jejunal or ileal atresia may be suspected antenatally based on the presence of hyperechoic, dilated bowel and polyhydramnios. It is not always possible to identify small bowel atresia antenatally and the presence of dilated bowel loops antenatally is not always associated with postnatal problems. In the neonatal period, infants may present with distension, bilious vomiting and failure to pass meconium; some infants, however, may pass meconium depending on timing of development of the atresia and so this does not exclude an atresia. Abdominal X-ray typically demonstrates significantly dilated proximal bowel loops, with the number of dilated loops relating to the level of obstruction (see Figure 5.3). A contrast enema may be performed demonstrating a small, unused colon (Microcolon) with the inability to reflux contrast into the dilated loops.

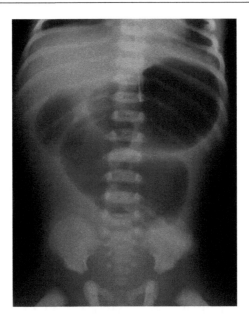

FIGURE 5.3   Abdominal radiograph of a neonate with proximal intestinal obstruction.

Operative management involves identification and resection of the atretic segment, any other atresia, as well as measurement of the bowel length. Formation of stomas or anastomosis, with or without tapering, may be appropriate with consideration to disparity in size between the two bowel ends. Total intestinal length must also be considered when determining surgical management, particularly when considering resection of the dilated proximal bowel. In general, the outcomes for patients with small bowel atresia are excellent as long as there is sufficient intestinal length to allow for enteral sufficiency. Very dilated or ectatic segments of bowel can cause problems with poor motility and impaired intestinal transit and it is important to plan for parenteral nutrition following neonatal surgery.

In patients in whom there has been no antenatal diagnosis of dilated bowel loops, it is probable that they will have been born in a local unit. After birth, they may present with poor feeding or feed refusal as well as bile-stained vomiting. Abdominal distension is a less common feature, and a subsequent abnormal plain radiograph often leads to referral. Care should be taken to decompress the stomach and proximal small bowel prior to aeromedical retrieval and careful liaison between neonatal retrieval services and paediatric surgery is essential to allow for appropriate planning of care. When an antenatal diagnosis of intestinal atresia is suspected, it is possible to plan more effectively and to talk to the family prior to delivery to allow them to prepare for potential medical treatment in the neonatal period. The following steps are recommended once a potential diagnosis of small bowel intestinal atresia is made:

- A discussion between the fetal medicine team/neonatal team/paediatric surgical team to plan for care following delivery.
- The family are offered antenatal counselling with a paediatric surgeon.
- Immediately after delivery, an NGT/OGT is placed to look for bile-stained aspirates.
- Feeds are withheld and a plain abdominal radiograph is taken after a few hours to determine the gas pattern.
- Further radiology can be organised to look for intestinal rotational anomalies or distal obstruction/microcolon.
- If the baby is stable and there is no abdominal tenderness, then a planned operation can take place in daylight hours to fix the intestinal atresia.

Colonic Atresia

Colonic atresia is seen uncommonly, representing less than 10% of intestinal atresia with an estimated incidence of around 1 in 20,000 live births. The aetiology and classification of colonic atresia is similar to that of ileo-jejunal atresia. Other congenital anomalies may be seen, with the association of Hirschsprung disease being of particular importance.

As a more distal obstruction, signs and symptoms such as distension and vomiting may develop later in the postnatal period than other atresia. X-ray findings may vary from multiple dilated bowel loops to a single large dilated colonic loop depending on the presence of a competent ileocaecal valve, with these infants also being at increased risk for perforation with a closed loop obstruction. A contrast enema can help confirm the diagnosis.

Operative management may include anastomosis or stoma formation. Primary anastomosis should, however, be approached with caution if Hirschsprung disease has not been excluded with a suction rectal biopsy prior to surgery. Although it is discussed here as part of the section on intestinal atresia, the clinical presentation and management have more in common with the other causes of distal intestinal obstruction [i.e. Hirschsprung disease, meconium ileus and anorectal malformation (ARM)].

ABNORMALITIES OF INTESTINAL ROTATION

The normal process of development of the gastrointestinal tract results in fixation of the bowel with the duodenojejunal flexure positioned to the left of the spine at the ligament of Treitz, the caecum fixed within the right lower quadrant with a broad-based mesentery between them, and the ascending and descending colon fixed in the retroperitoneum. During the embryonic period, the midgut forms a U-shaped loop which rapidly elongates and herniates through the umbilical cord during week 6 of gestation due to disproportionate growth. By week 10, the abdominal cavity has enlarged enough to allow return of the herniated loops. During this process, the midgut also undergoes a 270-degree rotation counter-clockwise around the axis of the superior mesenteric artery, resulting in the normal anatomy described earlier.

Failure at any stage of this process may result in a rotational anomaly. Complete non-rotation may occur, resulting in the duodenojejunal limb of the midgut sitting in the right abdomen and the caeco-colic limb on the left. Malrotation or incomplete rotation occurs when rotation is arrested at or near 180 degrees and typically results in the duodenojejunal flexure sitting the right of midline with the caecum in the upper abdomen and obstructing Ladd's bands across the duodenum. Reverse rotation due to rotation in a clockwise direction is rarely seen.

The significance of rotational anomalies lies in the width of the mesentery and subsequent risk of volvulus. In anomalies with a narrow-based mesentery, volvulus may occur with its potential catastrophic consequence of necrosis and loss of the entire midgut. A majority of cases of midgut volvulus in the setting of malrotation occur within the first month of life. Bilious vomiting may be the only initial sign in an infant with volvulus, and as such malrotation should be urgently excluded in all such presentations. Over time, the infant may develop further signs of intestinal ischaemia, necrosis or sepsis if untreated. Features of normal rotation on an upper gastrointestinal contrast study include a duodenojejunal flexure lying to the left of the spine, at the level of the pylorus, in a retroperitoneal position. Abnormality of any of these features is suggestive of a rotational anomaly, and in the setting of volvulus, a corkscrew appearance or 'beaking' of the duodenum may also be seen.

Surgical management of malrotation is undertaken by widening the mesentery, dividing any Ladd's bands and returning the bowel in a position of non-rotation with the small bowel on the right and colon on the left. **If there is any suspicion of volvulus, surgery should be performed emergently with detorsion of the volved midgut and assessment of viability**. In some cases, the entire midgut may be ischaemic or necrotic, resulting in short gut and potential lifelong need for TPN or transplant. In this scenario, a second-look laparotomy 24–48 hours following the first procedure may help guide management and allow further decision-making by the surgical and neonatal teams as well as the family. Appendicectomy may be performed as a component of the Ladd's procedure or left in situ to avoid conversion of an otherwise clean procedure to a contaminated one.

Malrotation with volvulus remains one of the most important conditions for paediatric surgeons. Timely diagnosis and initiation of management are essential in preventing intestinal insufficiency in an often otherwise healthy infant. The key feature of malrotation is **bile-stained vomiting**. The patient may also have demonstrated feed intolerance or been generally unsettled. By the time, physiological deterioration has occurred with a raised lactate and metabolic acidosis the position may already be irretrievable. Patients who have a suspected rotational abnormality remain a particular challenge in our geographically dispersed region. It is often not possible to organise radiological investigations to adequately exclude malrotation in smaller centres, and it is often necessary to transfer patients to a centre with both paediatric radiology and paediatric surgical expertise to facilitate management. In general, we would recommend the following steps for an infant with bile-stained vomiting:

- Immediate discussion with the paediatric surgical team.
- Fluid resuscitation is commenced where required.
- IV fluids and empiric antibiotics are initiated.
- Blood is taken for routine bloods and a capillary or venous gas sample is taken (including lactate where available).
- An NGT is placed and the stomach decompressed.
- A full physical examination is completed, including a rectal examination to look for blood PR.
- An abdominal radiograph is performed.
- Aeromedical retrieval is organised promptly.

It is important to emphasise that not all infants with bile-stained vomiting are subsequently diagnosed with a surgical pathology; however, malrotation with volvulus is difficult to exclude without further investigations and specialist assessment.

Meconium Ileus

Meconium ileus is a form of distal intestinal obstruction secondary to thickened, inspissated meconium, typically seen in infants with cystic fibrosis. Meconium ileus will be the presenting feature in up to 20% of children with cystic fibrosis and is rare in children without the disease. As such, all infants with meconium ileus should undergo careful investigation to confirm a diagnosis of cystic fibrosis. Dehydrated meconium (secondary to abnormal mucus secretion and enzyme deficiency) obstructs the terminal ileum in these infants, beginning in utero. Prenatal ultrasound may demonstrate dilated bowel loops as well as potential features of complications such as ascites. Postnatally, abdominal distension and development of bilious vomiting or aspirates may be noted, as well as failure to pass meconium. Meconium ileus may be classified as either simple (without features of complication), or complex with features such as segmental volvulus, bowel ischaemia and necrosis, atresia, or meconium peritonitis or pseudo-cyst secondary to perforation. Neonates with complex disease may be profoundly unwell and will present much earlier in life than those with simple meconium ileus, in some cases presenting at birth with significant abdominal distension and discolouration.

Management of these infants involves initial medical stabilisation with intravenous fluids, antibiotics and placement of a nasogastric tube. Abdominal X-ray may demonstrate dilated bowel loops, with or without air-fluid levels, as well as a ground glass or soap bubble appearance of the inspissated meconium. Where simple meconium ileus is suspected, performance of a contrast enema may be both diagnostic and therapeutic once the neonate has been adequately stabilised and resuscitated. Reflux of contrast into the dilated small bowel loops with characteristic filling defects secondary to the inspissated meconium helps confirm the diagnosis, as well as softening the meconium and potentially relieving the obstruction. A second attempt at a contrast enema may be considered if complete resolution is not achieved; however, in neonates where this is unsuccessful, or those with complicated disease, surgical management is indicated.

Operative intervention involves laparotomy, decompression of the obstructed bowel via enterotomy, and formation of a stoma or anastomosis in the scenario of simple disease. Adjuncts such as N-acetylcysteine may be useful in clearing the bowel of the thickened meconium. Administration postoperatively via nasogastric tube may also help with management of the thick gastrointestinal secretions. In complex disease, further management may be required, including control of sepsis and meconium peritonitis, resection of any necrotic or non-viable bowel, and management of intestinal atresia. Careful consideration should be given to the remaining bowel length and preserving viable bowel as far as possible.

A management plan for a patient with clinical features of distal intestinal obstruction is outlined next. In general, these patients do not present antenatally but rather with progressive abdominal distension and feed intolerance in an otherwise healthy infant. In the case of anorectal anomalies, physical examination may lead to a diagnosis being made, but in the case of Hirschsprung disease or meconium ileus, the diagnosis is often first made after an abnormal plain abdominal radiograph.

- A child with non-tender abdominal distension should have an NGT passed and feeds stopped.
- A plain radiograph should be performed urgently.
- A formal assessment by a neonatologist/paediatrician should ensure the child is appropriately resuscitated and IV access is established.
- If there are signs of distal obstruction, paediatric surgery should be consulted.
- Further investigations are then undertaken in a timely manner to look for causes of obstruction (e.g. a distal contrast study for suspected Meconium Ileus).
- The development of abdominal tenderness may indicate the need for urgent surgery.
- If the child is in a peripheral unit, they should be urgently retrieved to a centre where paediatric surgery/radiology and NICU are available.

Hirschsprung Disease

Hirschsprung disease, or colonic aganglionosis, is a congenital malformation defined by the absence of ganglion cells in the myenteric and submucosal plexuses of the terminal rectum, extending to a variable extent into the more proximal bowel. It affects around 1 in 5000 live births with an overall male predominance of 3–4:1; however, approaches equal sex distribution for total colonic disease.

During embryonic development, neural crest cells migrate through the gastrointestinal tract from proximal to distal and following this mature into ganglion cells. Theories of development of Hirschsprung disease therefore include failure of the neural crest cells to complete migration, failure of maturation, or failure of mature cells to survive or proliferate. Various genes have been implicated in the development of Hirschsprung disease, in particular, the RET proto-oncogene which is associated with familial and long-segment disease, and mutations in the endothelin family of genes which is associated with other neurocristopathies such as Waardenburg syndrome or congenital central hypoventilation syndrome.

Hirschsprung disease is not usually detected prenatally, with most cases being diagnosed in the neonatal period following development of features consistent with distal intestinal obstruction, i.e. abdominal distension, bilious vomiting and feed intolerance. **Delayed passage of meconium beyond the first 24 hours of life is a key feature and is seen in over 90% of cases**. Infants may occasionally present with perforation or Hirschsprung-associated enterocolitis (HAEC). Less commonly, diagnosis may be delayed beyond the neonatal period with children presenting with severe, chronic constipation and failure to thrive.

Investigation with abdominal X-ray may demonstrate dilated bowel loops throughout the abdomen with a paucity of distal gas. Contrast enema may be performed, with the pathognomonic finding being a transition zone between normal and aganglionic bowel. This may not, however, always be evident on contrast enema, and, in particular, with longer segment disease, the contrast study may not be diagnostic.

The gold standard for diagnosis is performance of a rectal biopsy, which in the neonatal period would typically be performed as a suction rectal biopsy in the neonatal unit. The diagnosis of Hirschsprung disease is made when no ganglion cells are identified in an adequate biopsy, with other features, including presence of hypertrophic nerves, abnormal acetylcholinesterase staining and absent expression of calretinin aiding in diagnosis.

Various surgical procedures have been described for the management of Hirschsprung disease with the goal of removing the aganglionic bowel to overcome obstruction whilst maintaining continence. Surgical approach may vary depending on the level of the transition zone between ganglionated and aganglionic bowel. In around 80%, the transition zone will be identified in the rectosigmoid region, with a further 10% having a more proximal transition zone within the colon and up to 10% total colonic aganglionosis.

The first described procedure for Hirschsprung disease, the Swenson procedure, involves resection of the aganglionic colon with formation of an anastomosis of ganglionated bowel just above the level of the sphincters. Due to concern about potential damage to vital pelvic structures with this technique, other procedures have emerged, including the Soave procedure where an aganglionic muscular cuff of rectum is left, and the Duhamel procedure where ganglionated bowel is brought down posterior to the rectum with formation of a stapled anastomosis. There is not, however, clear evidence of the superiority of any one technique.

Consideration should also be given to the risk of Hirschsprung-associated enterocolitis (HAEC) in these infants. Characterised by abdominal distension, fever and lethargy, and bloody stool or diarrhoea, early recognition and management of HAEC are vital with reported mortality of 1–10%, particularly in neonates. HAEC may be the presenting feature in some infants; however, risk of HAEC continues even after surgical intervention with removal of aganglionic bowel. Infants with long-segment disease and trisomy 21 appear to be at higher risk for development of HAEC. An approach to the child with suspected Hirschsprung disease is outlined below:

- Child presents with feed intolerance delayed passage of meconium and abdominal distension.
- Plain abdominal radiography performed.
- Feeds are ceased and IV access established IV fluids commenced.
- An NGT is passed and kept on free drainage.
- Complete physical examination performed.
- Paediatric surgery consulted.
- If abdomen tender or blood PR commence, IV antibiotics are given.
- A distal washout may be performed with warm saline to achieve decompression.
- Rectal examination may be followed by explosive and decompressive passage of stools and gas.
- Failure to decompress may result in urgent surgery to form a colostomy.
- Ideally, a diagnosis is confirmed with a suction rectal biopsy prior to surgery.
- A primary pull-through may be performed in selected neonates.

Anorectal Malformations

ARMs encompass a group of anatomic anomalies with maldevelopment of the anorectal region. The incidence of ARMs is around 1 in 5000 live births, with a male predominance.

Various classification systems have been utilised to define ARMs based on the level of the anomaly or presence and location of fistula. The Krickenbeck classification (2005) divided anomalies into two

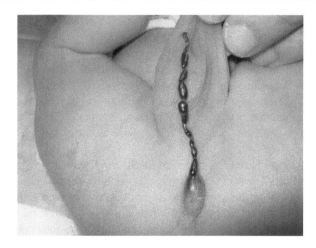

FIGURE 5.4   Make infant with imperforate anus and perineal fistula (low ARM).

groups: major clinical groups and rare or regional variants. Major clinical groups encompass perineal (cutaneous) fistula, recto-urethral fistula (prostatic or bulbar), recto-vesical fistula, recto-vestibular fistula, cloaca, no fistula and anal stenosis. Rare or regional variants include pouch colon, rectal atresia or stenosis, recto-vaginal fistula and H-type fistula. An example of a male infant with a perineal fistula can be seen in Figure 5.4. A more extreme example of ARM seen in females is cloaca and an image of a female infant with this condition can be seen in Chapter 13 (Figure 13.5).

Other associated anomalies may be seen, such as features of VACTERL, the association of trisomy 21 with imperforate anus without fistula or the Currarino triad in cases of anorectal stenosis (involvement of a pre-sacral mass and sacral anomalies in addition the ARM). Antenatal diagnosis is uncommon other than in cases of cloaca.

Postnatally, the absence of a normal anal opening may be noted on the newborn examination, along with potentially other features of VACTERL that may raise suspicion for the diagnosis. If the diagnosis and management is delayed, the infant may present with progressive distension and bilious aspirates or vomiting and may or may not pass meconium depending on the specific anatomy and location of a fistula. Presence of a fistula may not be immediately obvious in the first 24 hours until sufficient pressure has developed within the rectal pouch.

Initial management of the neonate with an ARM will depend on their ability to decompress via the fistula. In some variants, such as perineal fistula, recto-vestibular fistula or anal stenosis, adequate decompression may be achieved with gentle calibration using Hegar dilators. Some authors advocate for an early primary repair in these scenarios, whilst others would allow the neonate to be discharged and perform their repair at several months of age. In other types of ARM such as recto-urethral fistula or imperforate anus, the neonate will be unable to decompress and will require formation of a colostomy early in life. In this scenario, a high-pressure distal colostogram is vital in determining the anatomy and presence of a fistula prior to surgical planning.

The definitive surgical approach varies depending on the specific malformation. Many defects may be approached via a posterior sagittal anorectoplasty (PSARP). In the case of recto-vesical fistula, the rectum will not be able to be reached with a purely posterior sagittal approach, requiring both an abdominal (laparotomy or laparoscopy) and perineal approach.

Long-term outcomes in these children are variable. Children with lower malformations (for example perineal fistula or recto-vaginal fistula) tend to have better prognosis for continence, although they may have a tendency for constipation. Malformations such as recto-vesical or recto-prostatic urethral fistulas will have a more pessimistic prognosis in terms of their faecal continence. Consideration must also be given to the quality of the spine and the sacrum which will also influence longer-term outcomes, as described in the ARM Continence Index.

Cloaca, where the urinary tract, bowel and vagina join together in a common channel of variable length, represents a unique challenge. The distended, fluid-filled vagina or hemi-vagina may cause trigonal compression and obstruction of the urinary tract. Decompression may be attempted with catheter drainage, or formation of a vaginostomy at the time of colostomy formation. Long-term outcomes and reconstruction will be dependent on the length of the common channel. A common channel of less than 3 cm typically portends a better prognosis, with long common channels of greater than 3 cm portending worse outcomes in terms of bladder and bowel control as well as a far more complex reconstruction.

A summary of the initial management of a neonate with a suspected ARM is outlined in the following:

- Feeds should be stopped, and IV access established.
- An NGT/OGT should be placed the position checked and put on free drainage.
- Appropriate IV fluids should be given, and resuscitation commenced as clinically appropriate.
- IV antibiotics, including anaerobic cover, should be given.
- All babies should have IM/IV vitamin K given.
- A chest and abdominal plain radiograph should be taken.
- A complete physical examination should be performed looking for other anomalies (VACTERL).
- A paediatric surgeon should be consulted, and the patient should be retrieved to a centre with paediatric surgery/NICU/paediatric radiology availability.
- A urine specimen should be taken in male infants for microscopy to look for the presence of meconium.
- Although it may be possible to determine the level of obstruction clinically, further imaging is often required.

ABDOMINAL WALL DEFECTS

Gastroschisis

Gastroschisis consists of a full-thickness abdominal wall defect which is typically found to the right of the umbilicus. The eviscerated bowel is not covered with a membrane or sac and so is exposed to the amniotic fluid with subsequent bowel injury. Although uncommon, the incidence of this anomaly appears to be increasing over time, with an approximate incidence of 4–5 in 10,000 live births. As previously mentioned, the incidence in North Queensland appears to be higher at around 1:1000 live births. A picture of an infant with gastroschisis can be seen in Chapter 4 (Figure 4.1).

Unlike covered anterior abdominal wall defects, gastroschisis is not usually associated with other major congenital defects and usually occurs in isolation, although in male infants an association with undescended testes may be seen.

The aetiology of gastroschisis is not well understood, with multiple theories of embryological development, including a failure of mesoderm development in the body wall, abnormal involution of the right umbilical vein or disruption of the right vitelline artery, abnormal body wall folding, or failure of inclusion of yolk sac and vitelline structures within the body wall.

Gastroschisis is almost always diagnosed antenatally with evidence on ultrasound of a defect in the abdominal wall to the right of a normal umbilical cord, with extra-abdominal bowel loops not contained within a sac. Elevated maternal alpha feto-protein (AFP) is also seen. Delivery at a tertiary paediatric centre is recommended to avoid delay in management; however, there is no evidence to support any particular mode of delivery (caesarean or vaginal delivery) or preterm delivery.

Following delivery, the neonate with gastroschisis should have intravenous access established and administration of fluids. A nasogastric tube should be placed to decompress the stomach. Of key importance is inspection and protection of the exposed bowel. This can be achieved by wrapping of the bowel in cling film and placing it either in a central position on the abdomen supported by a 'doughnut' wrapping of dressings, or by placing the baby on the right side. It is vitally important to prevent kinking of the mesentery to avoid ischaemia to the bowel.

Management of these infants involves reduction of the eviscerated bowel to the abdominal cavity. This may be achieved primarily, or in infants where immediate reduction would lead to unacceptable intra-abdominal pressures via a staged approach with initial placement of the bowel within a silo followed by sequential reduction of the bowel over the following days. Methods of reduction and closure also differ, with some surgeons or centres undertaking this procedure under a general anaesthetic in the operating theatre, and others performing reduction at the bedside in the neonatal intensive care unit with sedation or analgesia. Similarly, the fascia of the abdomen may be approximated with sutures or a sutureless closure may be performed.

Gastroschisis may either be simple or complex (with associated bowel necrosis, perforation or atresia). The presence of complex features makes the management and prognosis of an infant with gastroschisis more difficult, necessitating bowel resection and formation of stomas or bowel anastomosis. Less commonly, 'vanishing gastroschisis' may be encountered, where closure or reduction of the defect size antenatally leads to ischaemia and loss of the herniated bowel and the long-term complications of short bowel syndrome.

The long-term prognosis of infants with gastroschisis is generally good in the absence of complex disease and vanishing gastroschisis. Complications seen in the short term may include NEC, abdominal compartment syndrome or ventilatory compromise and would complications such as infection or dehiscence. Longer-term complications are often related to the quality and length of the bowel, such as adhesional complications or short bowel syndrome.

Gastroschisis is one of the commonest antenatally detected conditions requiring neonatal surgery. Families are often helped by seeing the paediatric surgical team antenatally and adequate planning of delivery and subsequent care reduces complications and improves outcomes. The following key management strategies should be followed once a diagnosis is made:

- Following antenatal diagnosis, the case should be discussed with the fetal medicine/neonatal team/paediatric surgery.
- Families often find antenatal counselling with paediatric surgery helpful and reassuring.
- Delivery should be planned wherever possible although vaginal delivery is general thought to be advantageous.
- Delivery should be planned for a centre where paediatric surgery is available.
- Sometimes babies are delivered spontaneously prior to relocation and these patients should be resuscitated and stabilised locally and emergency transfer organised.
- The important factors in immediate resuscitation are to keep the baby 'warm, pink and sweet' (i.e. prevent hypothermia, oxygenate and maintain the bowel perfusion, and check the glucose).
- Feeds should be withheld.
- IV antibiotics should be given.
- IV fluids should be commenced and may need to be increased from standard infusion rates because of evaporative losses from uncovered bowel.
- An NGT should be placed, the position should be checked and it should be aspirated frequently to prevent gastric distension.
- The bowel can be covered with a non-occlusive dressing such as cling-film.
- The bowel should be supported to prevent kinking of mesenteric vessels.
- Reduction of the bowel may not require general anaesthesia and bedside silo application, or reduction is becoming more widely utilised.

Omphalocele

In contrast to gastroschisis, omphaloceles are true umbilical ring defects which are characterised by herniation of the abdominal viscera through the umbilicus. The defect is covered by a multi-layered membrane consisting of peritoneum, Wharton's jelly and amnion which protects the viscera from exposure to the amniotic fluid. The incidence of omphalocele is around 1 in 4000–6000 live births. A picture of an infant with exomphalos can be seen in Chapter 4 (Figure 4.2).

The aetiology and development of omphalocele are incompletely understood but thought to develop due to failure of body fold development (typically the lateral folds) resulting in a ventral abdominal wall defect of varying size. 'Giant' omphalocele is variably defined but may include defects larger than 5 cm or with herniation of the liver. Counter-intuitively, associated anomalies are seen frequently and more commonly with smaller defects. These include structural anomalies (such as cardiac, genitourinary, gastrointestinal, neural tube or diaphragmatic defects), chromosomal anomalies (including trisomies 13, 18 and 21 and Turner syndrome) and syndromes such as Beckwith–Weidemann and the Pentalogy of Cantrell. Omphalocele is typically diagnosed antenatally and due to the aforementioned associations karyotyping and fetal echocardiogram is recommended. Most pregnancies can be expected to deliver near term with no indication for preterm delivery. Small omphaloceles are typically able to safely deliver vaginally but larger defects containing liver generally require caesarean section due to the risk of sac rupture or liver injury.

Following delivery, the baby with omphalocele should be stabilised, with particular attention to the potential for significant pulmonary hypoplasia in large defects and need for respiratory support. The general condition of the baby and presence of any dysmorphic features should be considered as well as the degree of abdomino-visceral disproportion. Intravenous access should be established with the neonate commenced on fluids and antibiotics, and placement of a nasogastric tube for decompression. Hypoglycaemia must always be considered due to the association with Beckwith–Weidemann syndrome and so blood glucose levels should be monitored. Following stabilisation, further work-up for associated anomalies with an echocardiogram and renal ultrasound should be undertaken.

Management of omphalocele may vary significantly depending on the size of the defect and the presence of associated anomalies. An infant with a small defect and no significant abdomino-visceral disproportion may be suitable for primary closure of the defect early in the neonatal period. Larger defects with significant herniation of abdominal viscera, however, pose an ongoing challenge to appropriate management. Some authors have advocated for gradual serial reduction, similar to gastroschisis, using the sac itself or an artificial mesh or silo. Other techniques include painting or dressing of the sac with various topical agents to allow epithelialisation with repair of the large ventral hernia later in childhood. Survival in these infants is usually dictated by their associated anomalies, particularly major cardiac or chromosomal defects.

The initial management of covered abdominal wall defects can be summarised as follows:

- After a diagnosis is made antenatally, the patient should be discussed with fetal medicine/paediatric surgery/neonatology and a plan made for management after delivery.
- The family should be offered antenatal counselling with paediatric surgery.
- Other abnormalities and, in particular, chromosomal abnormalities should be looked for.
- Following delivery, the child should have an NGT placed.
- The child should not be fed until a detailed assessment is completed.
- IV access should be established, and IV fluids commenced.
- Care should be taken to look for hypoglycaemia and treat this appropriately.
- The size of the defect and clinical status of the neonate dictate subsequent management and surgical approach.

NECROTISING ENTEROCOLITIS

Necrotising enterocolitis (NEC) is the commonest condition requiring abdominal surgery in neonatal life. Various pathophysiological pathways lead to the clinical entity of NEC, with its final outcome of intestinal necrosis. NEC is seen in two groups of infants: premature neonates (classical NEC, responsible for more than 90% of cases) and term infants with co-morbidities such as congenital cardiac disease or haematological risk factors leading to poor mesenteric perfusion.

In premature infants, the aetiology of NEC is likely inflammatory, rather than ischaemic as in term infants, and involves an insult to the immature intestinal tract which triggers an exaggerated immune response in the setting of failure of protective factors. Significant maturation of the gastrointestinal tract and immune system occurs late in gestation, and as such the premature infant is predisposed to NEC due to their immature intestinal barrier and vasculature, lack of immunological defence and dysbiosis of the gut.

Other predisposing factors to the development of NEC in premature infants include commencement of enteral feeding, antibiotic use (which may decrease diversity of the intestinal micro-biome) and usage of medications which decrease gastric acid production (such as H2 antagonists). Protective factors include breast feeding, as breast milk contains multiple components that may be protective against infectious and inflammatory processes, as well as use of probiotics.

Diagnosis of NEC, particularly in the early stages, may be difficult as there can be significant overlap with other disease processes that may be seen in neonates such as spontaneous intestinal perforation, septic ileus or food protein intolerance. Early in the disease course, signs and symptoms may be subtle such as mild abdominal distension, apnoeic episodes and bradycardias, and temperature instability (stage I of the modified Bell staging criteria). With progression of disease, developments of bloody stools, thrombocytopenia and the pathognomonic finding of pneumatosis on abdominal X-ray help to establish the diagnosis and correlate with modified Bell stages II and III.

Initial medical management includes cessation of enteral feeds, decompression with placement of a nasogastric tube, administration of broad-spectrum antibiotics, cardio-respiratory support as required and regular reassessment of the infant. Evidence of perforation with pneumoperitoneum on abdominal X-ray is a definitive indication for surgical intervention, with relative indications, including failure of the baby to progress despite maximal medical management, presence of portal venous gas or persistence of a fixed bowel loop on serial imaging and examination. An example of a plain abdominal radiograph in a premature infant with extensive NEC can be seen in Figure 5.5.

Surgical management may involve initial placement of a peritoneal drain in the neonatal unit, or laparotomy with the aims of controlling sepsis and removing any frankly necrotic bowel. Assessment of the extent of disease should be performed with consideration of residual bowel length following resection. In the setting of limited, focal disease, resection of the necrotic or perforated segment with formation of stomas or in some settings primary anastomosis may be appropriate. Where disease is more extensive and resection would result in an unacceptably short length of remaining bowel, or if there are segments where potential viability is unclear, a re-look laparotomy in 48–72 hours may be indicated following resection of only areas of frank necrosis or perforation.

Necrotising enterocolitis totalis, with involvement of nearly the entire gut, is a rare but catastrophic form of NEC with significant mortality and consequences of short bowel syndrome and TPN reliance in surviving infants.

Longer-term, recurrent NEC or stricture formation may be seen, as well as the longer-term risks of neurodevelopmental complications. As our understanding of the disease process and underlying aetiological factors develops, these outcomes may also continue to improve.

The underlying pathogenesis of NEC is poorly understood. In general, neonates with this condition are often premature with significant other problems of prematurity and so it is most common for these

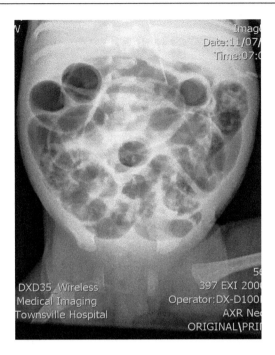

FIGURE 5.5   Abdominal radiograph of a neonate with necrotising enterocolitis.

patients to be referred by the neonatal team in a tertiary-level centre to paediatric surgery rather than necessitating transfer. The principal steps in the management of NEC are initially supportive by the neonatal team and as such lie outside the scope of this chapter. In general, the commonest approach is to rest the intestine and treat with parenteral antibiotics and support the neonate with TPN. Often supportive measures lead to a gradual improvement in the clinical situation without the need for surgery. However, it is important to consult with paediatric surgery as early as possible in the disease course to allow for planning should deterioration occur. This allows for early contact with the family to help establish rapport as well as allowing for serial examination to determine those patients who are not progressing to recovery as we would expect. A brief outline of the management of the neonate with suspected NEC is outlined in the following:

- Commence resuscitation and try to stabilise physiological parameters.
- Check FBC/WCC/platelets look for metabolic acidosis and lactate.
- Stop feeds and place NGT on free drainage, aspirate frequently particularly if ventilated.
- Perform serial plain abdominal radiography to look for signs of pneumatosis intestinalis and to exclude perforation.
- Commence IV fluids and TPN as well as parenteral antibiotics.
- A stool test for calprotectin may help support a diagnosis of NEC in some cases.
- Serial and regular abdominal examination should be performed to look for signs of perforation/development of a mass/fixed loop or abdominal tenderness.
- A failure to demonstrate improvement or progression of disease is indications to consider laparotomy.
- Prior to surgery, blood should be requested and clotting checked.

SUMMARY

Neonatal surgery remains a challenge for paediatric surgeons. The best results are achieved when planning with a number of teams is commenced prior to the need for surgery. Many conditions are diagnosed antenatally providing us with the opportunity to inform and reassure families as well as to allow for planning of management prior to delivery. This is particularly important for families who may reside in rural and remote locations where there is usually no access to specialist paediatric surgical or NICU services.

Whilst the challenges in managing these conditions are large, the outcomes for these patients continue to improve, and for the large majority of patients, the outcomes are excellent. A systematic approach involving stabilisation and resuscitation, planning and communication are essential components in successful management. Wherever possible transfer should take place prior to delivery and in cases where this has not been possible careful planning should be made to ensure the least physiological disturbance during aeromedical transfer. We are fortunate to have specialised neonatal retrieval services but for those surgeons without access to these teams then careful communication with local healthcare providers is almost always beneficial.

A large number of neonatal surgical conditions have not been covered in this chapter, e.g. neonatal tumours, cystic hygroma as these are less common, but in general the same principles of early diagnosis, effective communication between teams and resuscitation and stabilisation remain important in successful management. Of the conditions we have discussed, neonatal lung lesions usually do not require emergency surgery (with the exception of CLE), neonatal intestinal problems, however, often require emergent surgery and management. These can be conveniently subdivided into proximal and distal intestinal obstruction for management purposes and the history and clinical examination along with simple plain abdominal radiography are often helpful in distinguishing between the different causes of intestinal obstruction.

Bile-stained vomiting is the single most important sign of surgical pathology and the consideration of malrotation and volvulus is mandated in babies with this sign. Failure to recognise this remains a significant cause of avoidable morbidity and mortality in otherwise healthy children.

FURTHER READING

Bruch SW, Langer JC. Omphalocele and gastroschisis. In: Puri P, editor. Newborn Surgery. 4th Edition. CRC Press; 2017.

Escobar MA, Caty MG. Meconium disease. In: Holcomb GW, Murphy JP, St Peter SD, editors. Holcomb and Ashcraft's Pediatric Surgery. 7th Edition. Elsevier Inc.; 2020.

Harting MT, Hollinger LE, Lally KP. Congenital diaphragmatic hernia and eventration. In: Holcomb GW, Murphy JP, St Peter SD, editors. Holcomb and Ashcraft's Pediatric Surgery. 7th Edition. Elsevier Inc.; 2020.

Javid PJ, Riggle KM, Smith C. Necrotizing enterocolitis. In: Avery's Diseases of the Newborn. 10th Edition. Elsevier Inc.; 2018.

Kieran EA, O'Donnell CPF. Specific risks for the preterm infant. In: Puri P, editor. Newborn Surgery. 4th Edition. CRC Press; 2017.

Laje P, Flake AW. Congenital bronchopulmonary malformations. In: Holcomb and Ashcraft's Pediatric Surgery. 7th Edition. Elsevier Inc.; 2020.

Langer JC. Hirschsprung disease. In: Holcomb GW, Murphy JP, St Peter SD, editors. Holcomb and Ashcraft's Pediatric Surgery. 7th Edition. Elsevier Inc.; 2020.

Losty PD. Esophageal atresia and tracheo-esophageal fistula. In: Newborn Surgery. 4th Edition. CRC Press; 2017.

Millar AJW, Numanoglu A, Cox S. Jejunoileal atresia and stenosis. In: Newborn Surgery. 4th Edition. CRC Press; 2017.

Millar AJW, Rode H, Cywes S. Malrotation and volvulus in infancy and childhood. Semin Pediatr Surg. 2003 November;12(4):229–36.

Ogle SB, Nichol PF, Ostlie DJ. Duodenal and intestinal atresia and stenosis. In: Holcomb GW, Murphy JP, St Peter SD, editors. Holcomb and Ashcraft's Pediiatric Surgery. 7th Edition. Elsevier Inc.; 2020.

Puri P, Tomuschat C. Hirschsprung's disease. In: Newborn Surgery. 4th Edition. CRC Press; 2017.

Rentea RM, Levitt MA. Anorectal atresia and cloacal malformations. In: Holcomb GW, Murphy JP, St Peter SD, editors. Holcomb and Ashcraft's Pediatric Surgery. 7th Edition. Elsevier Inc.; 2020.

Singh R, Davenport M. The argument for operative approach to asymptomatic lung lesions. Semin Pediatr Surg. 2015 August;24(4):187–9.

The Infant as a Paediatric Surgical Patient

6

Kapilan Ravichandran and Daniel Carroll

INTRODUCTION

The term infant is applied to very young children under 1 year of age. Infants have distinct surgical conditions and they should be expediently identified and corrected through both non-surgical and surgical interventions. This chapter will discuss the following: Inguinal hernia, intussusception, pyloric stenosis, tongue-tie, vascular anomalies and tropical skin infections, including kerion.

INGUINAL HERNIAS

A hernia is defined as an abnormal protrusion of an organ or tissue through a defect in its surrounding walls. In infancy, it is most common to see inguinal and umbilical hernias. An inguinal hernia in an infant is almost always an indirect inguinal hernia and requires urgent referral to a paediatric surgeon.

History

Over 400 years ago, Ambroise Pare described the reduction of an incarcerated inguinal hernia and the application of a truss. He recognised that inguinal hernias in children were probably congenital in nature and that they could be cured.

Anatomy

The inguinal canal is a passage in the anterior abdominal wall. It extends from the deep inguinal ring to the superficial inguinal ring. The deep inguinal ring lies at the mid-inguinal point just above the inguinal ligament. The margins of the ring are:

- *Inferiorly*: The inguinal ligament and medially the lacunar ligament
- *Medially*: The transversalis fascia
- *Superiorly and laterally*: The transversus abdominis

DOI: 10.1201/9781003156659-6

The contents of the inguinal canal are different in the male and the female. In the male, the contents of the inguinal canal are:

- The spermatic cord
- The cremaster muscle
- The Ilioinguinal nerve

The spermatic cord has seven components:

- Vas deferens
- Artery to the vas deferens
- Testicular artery
- Cremasteric artery
- Testicular veins
- Genital branch of the genitofemoral nerve
- Autonomic nerves

In the female, the contents of the inguinal canal are the round ligament and the ilioinguinal nerve.

It is important to remember that at birth the superficial and deep rings lie virtually on top of one another. As a child grows, the inguinal canal lengthens and it is approximately 4 cm in a fully grown adult.

Pathogenesis

Before birth, the layers of the processus vaginalis normally fuse, closing off the entrance to the inguinal canal from the abdominal cavity. It is common for the processus vaginalis to close incompletely, particularly in premature male infants. When luminal obliteration fails to occur, a sac is present into which abdominal contents may herniate if the defect at the internal ring is large enough. Even when the processus vaginalis is patent, the entrance may be adequately covered by the internal oblique and transverse abdominal muscles, preventing the escape of abdominal contents until later in childhood. It is clear that a spectrum of presentations from a hydrocoele of the cord to a large inguinoscrotal indirect hernia can be seen depending upon the size of the defect.

Epidemiology

The exact incidence of indirect inguinal hernia is unknown. Based on large series of patients, the incidence of inguinal hernia undergoing repair is around 5%. Males are more commonly affected than females with a male:female ratio of around 8–10:1.

Prematurity is associated with an increased incidence of inguinal hernias. Reported incidences as high as 30% have been presented in male infants.

Rarely some conditions are associated with an increased risk of inguinal hernias and an increased risk of recurrence after inguinal herniotomy:

- Cystic fibrosis
- Connective tissue disorders
- Mucopolysaccharidosis
- Congenital diaphragmatic hernia
- Peritoneal dialysis
- Patients with a ventriculoperitoneal shunt

DIRECT INGUINAL HERNIAS

Direct inguinal hernias are rare and tend not to be diagnosed preoperatively. Up to one-third of patients with a direct hernia or a femoral hernia have had a previous indirect inguinal hernia operation.

Clinical Presentation

The typical presentation is of a child with a groin swelling that in the male infant extends towards the top of the scrotum. It is most pronounced during episodes of increased intra-abdominal pressure, e.g. when crying. It often reduces spontaneously.

On clinical examination, there is a swelling originating at the site of the deep ring that extends a variable length towards the scrotum. It is not uncommon for a patient to be referred for a history suggestive of an inguinal hernia but for no hernia to present at the time of consultation. In these cases, palpation of a thickened cord over the pubic tubercle (silk glove sign) may be present, but sometimes it is necessary to operate on the basis of a consistent history alone. An example of a male infant with a right inguinal hernia can be seen in Figure 6.1.

Investigations

The majority of patients with an inguinal hernia can be diagnosed easily without the need for further investigation. It is not uncommon, however, for patients to be referred on the basis of an ultrasound scan (USS) demonstrating an abnormality in the inguinal canal. Generally, ultrasound scanning is useful only for carefully selected cases where the remains doubt after careful clinical assessment.

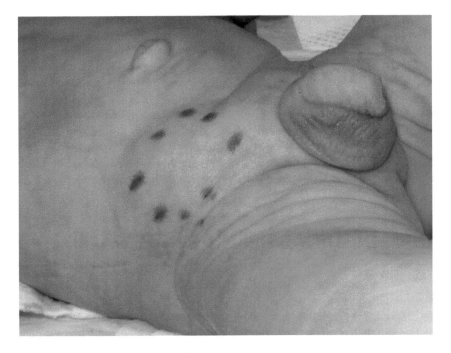

FIGURE 6.1   Infant male with a right inguinal hernia.

Management

Once a patient has been diagnosed with an inguinal hernia, surgery should be planned. The urgency of surgery is dependent upon the age of the child at the time of presentation with a hernia. The smaller the child when the hernia is first noted, the greater the risk of incarceration and strangulation. In remote settings, it is important to try and assess and fix a hernia wherever possible to reduce the risk of the need for urgent or emergency transfer to another centre.

In general, we recommend that children who are diagnosed with a hernia whilst neonates have these fixed prior to discharge from hospital. Those that are under a month of age at presentation should be fixed on the next available list and children over this age should be seen and assessed urgently and plans are made for admission and repair within 30 days. The parents should be told what to look for in case the hernia becomes incarcerated in the interim and what actions they should take (i.e. go to hospital).

On rare occasions, a child may present with a hernia that is incarcerated or even strangulated. In such instances, the patient should be resuscitated as necessary with the establishment of IV access and initiation of fluids as required. Parenteral antibiotics should be administered and the most experienced clinician available should attempt manual reduction of the hernia after the administration of appropriate pain relief. These patients often require transfer to paediatric surgical centres even if reduction is successful and the basic principles of safe transfer outlined previously should be followed. There is a significant risk of subsequent testicular atrophy in males (up to 50%) or damage to the ovary in females with obstructed, irreducible indirect inguinal hernias.

Operative Management

Inguinal herniotomy is carried out as a day case in the majority of cases. Premature infants and those patients with a corrected postnatal age of less than 1 month require inpatient observation following surgery because of the risk of apnoea. In the case of infants born prematurely, for every week of prematurity, 2 weeks should be added to their corrected age before they do not require admission and observation. A detailed description of the operation is beyond the scope of this chapter; however, it is important for any doctor taking consent for a procedure should be able to explain the basic steps of the procedure.

Once the child has been anaesthetised, positioned, prepped and draped then an incision is made over the lower border of external oblique between the internal and external rings. This is conveniently marked by a skin crease and the intersection of this skin crease and a line drawn directly upwards from the femoral pulse is a good surface marking for the location of the deep inguinal ring. The scrotum should be prepped and remain visible throughout the procedure. Once the skin and Scarpa's fascia have been opened, it is important to demonstrate the lower border of external oblique and identify the superficial ring prior to proceeding. It is then usual to open external oblique in a controlled fashion and deliver the cord. The vas and vessels are then gently dissected away from the hernial sac and a herniotomy is performed. The proximal end of the sac is transfixed with a dissolvable suture and external oblique is closed. At the end of the procedure, it is important to ensure and document that both testes are present within the scrotum.

INGUINAL HERNIAS IN FEMALES

Apart from the obvious anatomical differences, a significant number of inguinal hernias contain adnexal structures (ovary or fallopian tubes) (around 20%).

The initial approach in the female is identical to that in a male. Care must be taken when delivering the sac as traction can deliver adnexal structures complicating the procedure. Many surgeons choose to open the sac once it has been controlled to ensure that there are no adnexal structures present. On very rare occasions, a testis may appear during the repair. This is because the infant has male chromosomes but complete androgen insensitivity. At this point, it is important to contact the family and specialist paediatric teams prior to taking a biopsy of the abnormal a gonad and completing the herniotomy.

Laparoscopy

Over recent years, laparoscopy has been increasingly used in the management of inguinal hernias in children. The basic operative approach has been to ligate the processus vaginalis at the neck of the sac by partially closing the internal ring. In general, it is not used as a first-line approach although it is becoming more common, it is particularly useful for recurrent hernias.

Anaesthesia for Inguinal Hernia Repair

Most hernia repairs are performed under general anaesthetic. It is useful to be able to perform hernia repairs under spinal anaesthesia in selected infants, particularly those with chronic lung disease and prematurity as it reduces the postoperative risk of apnoea.

Summary and Key Points

- Inguinal hernias are common.
- Incarceration of a hernia occurs most frequently in infants (70%).
- Management depends upon the age of the child and the presentation.
- Emergency surgery is reserved for patients with irreducible hernias.
- Urgent surgery is planned for small infants.

INTUSSUSCEPTION

Intussusception refers to the invagination of a part of the intestine into itself. It is the most common cause of bowel obstruction in infants. Most cases in children are idiopathic and pathological lead points are identified in only 25% of cases involving children. This is divergent to adults where in the majority a pathological cause is identified.

Pathophysiology

In intussusception, the proximal bowel (intussusceptum) invaginates or telescopes inside the adjacent distal bowel (intussucipiens) by peristalsis. As it develops, the mesentery of the proximal bowel is drawn into the distal bowel, resulting in venous and lymphatic congestion with consequent intestinal oedema. If left untreated, arterial insufficiency occurs with subsequent ischaemia, perforation and peritonitis.

Primary Intussusception

Seventy-five per cent of cases of childhood intussusception are idiopathic as there is no pathological lead point. Idiopathic intussusception is most common in children between 3 months and 5 years. In such cases, the apex of the intussusception is most likely an area of enlarged submucosal lymphoid tissue – Peyer's patches in the distal ileum which has undergone reactive hyperplasia. Viral respiratory illness and gastroenteritis have been implicated as a preceding cause of hypertrophied lymphoid tissue. Approximately 30% of patients experience viral illness (URTI, otitis media, coryzal symptoms) before onset. A prospective case-control study examining infection triggers for intussusception in Vietnam and Australia, infection with adenovirus, species C emerged as the strongest predictor of intussusception in both populations, suggesting a strong association with adenovirus infection. The early form of the vaccine (RRV-TV: Rotashield) was removed from the market because of a 22-fold increase in intussusception among vaccinated infants. Bacterial enteritis is also associated with intussusception in which most cases occur within the first month of diagnosis. This association was noted for infection with *Salmonella*, *Escherichia coli*, *Shigella* or *Campylobacter*.

Secondary Intussusception

Secondary intussusception is where an identifiable lead point or variation in the intestine is trapped by peristalsis and thus draws the proximal bowel into the distal bowel. In 25% of cases, an underlying disease causing a pathological lead point is identified, accounting for a greater proportion with increasing age. The most common lead point is Meckel's diverticulum. Other causes include polyps and duplication cysts. Other benign lead points include the appendix, haemangiomas, carcinoid tumours, foreign bodies, ectopic pancreas or gastric mucosa, hamartomas from Peutz–Jeghers syndrome and lipomas. Malignant causes are rare but are likely to be lymphoma and small bowel tumours. Systemic diseases, such as Henoch–Schonlein purpura where a small bowel haematoma acts as a lead point or cystic fibrosis where thick inspissated stool may act as a lead point, have been associated with intussusception. Coeliac disease has also been implicated, with the pathogenesis related to dysmotility, excessive secretions and bowel wall weakness.

Classification

Intussusception is classified by its location. Ileocolic intussusception involves the ileocecal junction and accounts for 90% of all cases. Ileo-ileal, ileo-ileo-colic, jejuno-jejunal, jejuno-ileal or colo-colic have been described.

Incidence

The highest incidence occurs in infants between ages 4 and 9 months and typical presents between 3 and 36 months old. Ninety per cent of affected patients are younger than 2 years old. Approximately two-thirds of cases are boys.

Clinical Manifestation

Classical presentation in infants includes sudden intermittent, cramping, progressive abdominal pain, accompanied by inconsolable crying and drawing up of legs towards the abdomen, often with pallor. Episodes last between 15- and 20-minute intervals. Attacks of pain commence and cease abruptly and between attacks may appear comfortable. Vomiting is a prominent symptom and may be initially non-bilious, but as the obstruction progresses, it will become bilious. Stools will have occult blood in 25% and are grossly bloody in 50% of cases. The classical red currant jelly stools are a late sign as bowel wall ischaemia is what causes mucosal sloughing and compression of mucous glands leading to the evacuation of currant jelly stools. As symptoms progress, increasing lethargy often develops. The classically described triad of pain, palpable sausage-shaped mass, and red currant jelly stools are seen in less than 15% of patients at presentation.

Examination

If obstructive process worsens, and bowel ischaemia occurs, dehydration, fever, tachycardia and hypotension can develop in quick succession because of bowel ischaemia and consequent bacteraemia. There may be audible peristaltic rushes, and a sausage-shaped mass palpable is present anywhere in the abdomen, which is most commonly found in the right hypochondrium. The right lower abdominal quadrant can appear flat or empty (Dance's sign) as the intussusception is drawn cephalad. On rectal examination, blood-stained mucus or blood may be encountered as a later sign.

Differential Diagnosis

- Meckel's diverticulum
- Bacterial or amoebic colitis
- Malrotation with midgut volvulus
- Appendicitis
- Mesenteric ischaemia
- Ovarian torsion
- Incarcerated hernia

Diagnosis

Abdominal X-ray

The main purpose of the erect and supine abdominal radiograph is to exclude perforation, if present the patient requires operative management rather than non-operative reduction. Plain radiographs cannot be used to exclude intussusception particularly in patients in whom there is a high clinical suspicion of intussusception. The sensitivity for abdominal radiographs is less than 48%, while specificity is 21%. Suggestive abnormalities on radiography include signs of intestinal obstruction, crescent sign – soft tissue density (representing the intussusceptum) projecting into gas of the large bowel and lack of air in the caecum.

Ultrasonography

The sensitivity and specificity of US in detecting intussusception is 97.9% and 97.8%, respectively, in experienced ultrasonographers. Negative predictive value is 99.7% when the examination is performed by an experienced ultrasonographer. US detects pathological lead points and can be used to monitor the success of reduction procedure and does not expose patients to radiation. Furthermore, it can be used to evaluate for alternate causes for a patient's symptoms. The characteristic finding on US is referred to as a "target sign", which consists of alternating rings of low and high echogenicity representing the telescoping bowel wall and mesenteric fat within the intussusceptum transversely. Colour dopplers may reveal a lack of perfusion in the intussusceptum indicating the development of ischaemia. The possibility of small bowel intussusception rather than ileocolic intussusception increased when by the location of the intussusception is outside of the right lower quadrant.

Management

Non-operative management

Non-operative reduction using hydrostatic or pneumatic pressure by enema is the treatment of choice for an infant or child with ileocolic intussusception who is clinically stable. Contraindications include intestinal perforation, peritonitis or shocked state. The advantages of non-operative reduction are decreased morbidity, cost and length of hospitalisation.

Prior to reduction by enema, the patient should be stabilised and bowel rest and intravenous fluid resuscitation should be initiated. A nasogastric tube may be utilised to decompress the stomach. Full blood count and electrolytes are obtained. There is no requirement for prophylactic intravenous antibiotics prior to or during non-operative reduction except for children who are clinically unstable.

Hydrostatic and Pneumatic Reduction

Either the pneumatic or hydrostatic (saline or contrast) technique is acceptable for the reduction of intussusception in stable children. Pneumatic reduction is associated with a higher success rate of 83% compared to 70% for hydrostatic reduction. However, both methods have comparable rates of perforation and early recurrence. The standard method of hydrostatic reduction is to place a reservoir of fluid of 1 meter above the patient, so constant hydrostatic pressure is generated. Due to potential hazard of barium peritonitis, most institutions have transitioned to water-soluble isotonic contrast. Pneumatic technique begins with the insertion of a Foley catheter or rectal tube into the rectum with a tight seal. The procedure is fluoroscopically monitored as air is insufflated into the rectum. A sphygmomanometer can be used to monitor colonic intraluminal pressure to aid in reduction. Successful reduction is indicated by reflux of air into the terminal ileum, drop of intraluminal pressure and disappearance of mass. Non-operative reduction is successful in approximately 85% of patients and more likely to be achieved in patients with idiopathic intussusception. In some centres ultrasound guided hydrostatic reduction is performed using warmed saline rather than water-soluble contrast.

The main risk of hydrostatic or pneumatic reduction is perforation of the bowel which is reported as less than 1%. Perforation occurs on the distal side of intussusception often in the transverse colon. Tension pneumoperitoneum is treated with the cessation of procedure and the release of pneumoperitoneum as it can compromise the respiratory status of the patient. Hydrostatic and pneumatic reduction is less likely to be successful if there are symptoms present for greater than 24 hours and in older children with established small bowel obstruction.

Surgery

An operation is indicated when non-operative reduction is unsuccessful, in the presence of widespread peritonism, or when there is the presence of a pathological lead point or pneumoperitoneum. Preoperative preparation includes administration of broad-spectrum antibiotics, intravenous fluid resuscitation, insertion of a urinary catheter, and placement of a nasogastric tube for gastric decompression. Most laparoscopic approaches utilise three abdominal ports: One in the infraumbilical region, with two other ports along the left side of the abdomen. Reduction is completed through gentle pressure distal to the intussusceptum using atraumatic graspers. Traction is usually required proximal to the intussusceptions to complete the reduction which is divergent to the open approach. Risks factors for conversion to an open procedure include an intussusceptum extending beyond the ascending colon as well as presence of known pathologic lead points. Appendectomy is not routinely performed with laparoscopic or open reduction unless the appendix is a lead point.

Open approach is through a laparotomy via a transverse right supra-umbilical incision which allows delivery of the intussusceptum and it is gently manipulated back towards its normal position in the terminal

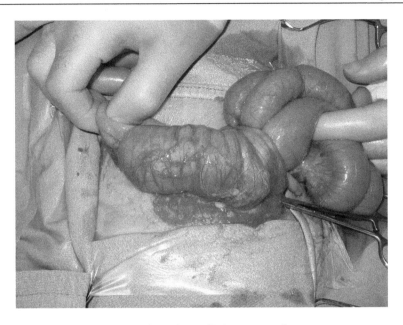

FIGURE 6.2   Intra-operative photograph of an oleo-colic intussusception.

ileum. The inability to reduce ischaemic bowel or the identification of a lead point requires resection and if possible primary anastomosis or diversion. A photograph of a laparotomy for ileo-colic intussusception is shown in Figure 6.2.

RECURRENT INTUSSUSCEPTION

Intussusception recurs more commonly after hydrostatic or pneumatic reduction than after surgery. It usually occurs within 2–3 days of the reduction.

The key points in the management of intussusception are summarised next:

- **If intussusception is suspected, resuscitation should be performed prior to obtaining radiological confirmation**.
- IV access should be established.
- The patient should be kept nil by mouth (NBM).
- A good-sized NGT should be placed to allow adequate drainage of the stomach.
- The patient should be monitored and given supplemental oxygen if required.
- The surgical team should be informed and be present prior to any attempted reduction.
- A fluid bolus and IV antibiotics should be given prior to attempting reduction.
- Pain relief should be given prior to attempting air reduction.
- This is typically with morphine so the child will require monitoring during and after attempted reduction.
- The surgical team should be prepared for the potential perforation during the procedure and available to perform needle decompression in such an event.
- Theatres and the anaesthetic team should be informed of the case prior to attempting either pneumatic or hydrostatic reduction.

RECTAL PROLAPSE

Rectal prolapse is common in young children and usually does not come to the attention of the paediatric surgeon. It most commonly occurs in the context of straining due to chronic constipation but can also be the presenting feature of diarrheal illnesses, malnutrition, wasting illnesses and most importantly (but rarely) cystic fibrosis. Prolapse is usually a herniation of the rectum through a dilated levator mechanism.

Three different clinical entities may coexist:

- Mucosal prolapse (partial or pseudoprolapse)
- Internal prolapse (rectal intussusception)
- Full-thickness rectal prolapse (complete or true)

It is the full-thickness rectal prolapse that often presents as an emergency. It is possible for a full-thickness rectal prolapse to become incarcerated and irreducible even resulting in strangulation of the rectum.

Management

In the case of an emergency presentation, it is important to reduce the rectal prolapse by inserting a finger into the rectum This also allows for the opportunity to examine to rule out an intussusception of the sigmoid colon. They usually resolve spontaneously. In the case of irreducible rectal prolapse, the patient should be transferred urgently to a paediatric surgical centre for ongoing management.

Treatment Options

The mainstay of treatment is to treat underlying constipation and voiding disorders by reducing the need for straining at stool. The conservative approach to manage such conditions is beyond the scope of this chapter. Surgical therapy has taken a number of forms, mostly unsatisfactory in their outcomes. Most commonly sclerotherapy with hypertonic saline is injected in the retrorectal space to produce an inflammatory response. This is performed under a general anaesthetic. This may need to be coupled with transanal suture fixation of the rectum.

HYPERTROPHIC PYLORIC STENOSIS

Infanftile hypertrophic pyloric stenosis (IHPS) is the most common cause of vomiting that requires surgical intervention. The reported incidence is 1:300 children, although this seems to be decreasing for unknown reasons. The incidence in Tropical North Queensland is markedly lower than this with an incidence around 1:2000. The cause for this is unknown.

Pathophysiology

The hallmark of pyloric stenosis is marked hypertrophy and hyperplasia of both the circular and longitudinal muscular layers of the pylorus. This thickening leads to the narrowing of the lumen of the gastric antrum and lengthening of pyloric canal, ultimately resulting in a gastric outlet obstruction.

Aetiology

The aetiology of IHPS is likely multifactorial with environmental influences. A genetic predisposition has been inferred from race discrepancies – more common in Caucasian infants as well as male predisposition – 4:1 male-to-female ratio. Variants near several loci, including *MBNL1, NKX2-5* and *APOA1*, have been associated with IHPS. Environmental factors associated with IHPS include the method of feeding (breast vs formula), seasonal variability, exposure to erythromycin, environmental pesticides and transpyloric feeding in premature infants.

Differential Diagnosis

- Gastro-oesophageal reflux disease (GORD)
- Gastroenteritis
- Increased intracranial pressure
- Antral web
- Foregut duplication cyst
- Gastric tumours
- Tumour causing extrinsic gastric compression

Clinical Manifestations

The classical presentation is non-bilious projectile vomiting in an otherwise well neonate who is between 2 and 8 weeks old. Initially the emesis is infrequent; however, over time, the emesis occurs post every feed. The contents of the emesis are usually recent feedings which often appear as curdled milk. Owing to gastritis secondary to gastric outlet obstruction, there can sometimes be a coffee ground vomitus. Initially, the child is active and hungry and a key feature is their readiness and ability to feed immediately vomiting. However, with increasing dehydration and electrolyte imbalance, the patient becomes progressively more somnolent and lethargic.

Examination

Careful assessment of the dehydration status should be completed. Pathognomonic examination finding is the palpation of the thickened pylorus, which on examination is akin to an olive. It is palpated most easily in a relaxed patient. After palpating the liver edge, the examiner's fingertips should slide underneath the liver in the midline. Then the examiner's fingers are pulled back down, trying to trap the "olive". When difficulty is experienced in feeling the tumour, a nasogastric tube is passed to decompress the stomach. If the hypertrophied pylorus cannot be palpated, US evaluation should be pursued. Owing to the profound metabolic disturbances which arise, full blood count, electrolytes and blood gas must be obtained on initial presentation.

Ultrasound

US has become the standard technique for diagnosing IHPS. The diagnostic criteria for pyloric stenosis are a muscle thickness of ≥4 mm and a pyloric length of ≥16 mm. A thickness of >3 mm is considered positive if the neonate is younger than 30 days of age. If the US findings are equivocal, then an upper

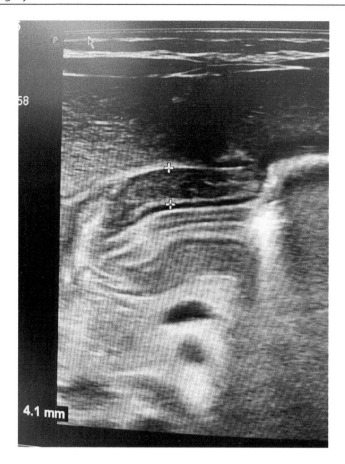

FIGURE 6.3   Ultrasound scan demonstrating pyloric stenosis.

gastrointestinal series can be helpful in confirming the diagnosis in which a "string sign" is indicative of IHPS. An example of a single image from a US examination of the pylorus in an infant with IHPS is seen in Figure 6.3.

Management

Initial management involves the correction of fluid and metabolic derangement. The hallmark metabolic derangement of hypochloremic, hypokalemic metabolic alkalosis is usually seen to some degree in most patients. There are numerous resuscitation protocols and involvement of the local paediatric team is paramount to peri-operatively optimise the infant. An expert panel recommended that laboratory values be normalised to at least the following thresholds prior to pyloromyotomy: pH ≤7.45, base excess ≤3.5, bicarbonate <26 mmol/L, sodium ≥132 mmol/L, potassium ≥3.5 mmol/L, chloride ≥100 mmol/L and glucose ≥4.0 mmol/L (72 mg/dL). Electrolytes should be checked every 6 hours until they normalise and the alkalosis has resolved. Pyloric stenosis is not a surgical emergency and resuscitation is of priority. Inadequate resuscitation can lead to postoperative apnoea due to decreased respiratory drive secondary to alkalosis.

Pyloromyotomy can be performed with either an open or laparoscopic approach. In the open approach, a right upper quadrant transverse incision was originally described, however it is now more usual to perform the operation via an omega-shaped incision around the umbilicus. The pylorus is exteriorised

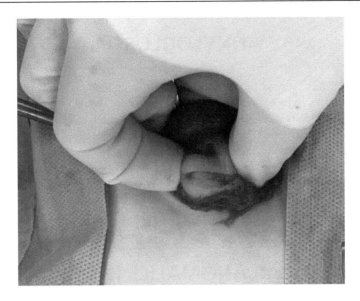

FIGURE 6.4   Operative photograph of open pyloromyotomy.

through the incision then a longitudinal serosal incision is made in the pylorus approximately 2 mm proximal to the junction of the duodenum and is carried onto the anterior gastric wall for approximately 5 mm. Blunt dissection is used to divide the firm pyloric fibres down to the submucosa. The pyloromyotomy is then completed by ensuring that all fibres are divided throughout the entire length of the incision. This is confirmed by visualising the circular muscle of the stomach proximally as well as a protrusion of the submucosa. The surgical principles are similar to a laparoscopic approach which has the added advantage of reduced length of stay as well as no difference in complication rates between the two approaches. After division, a small amount of gas from the stomach is passed through the pylorus to ensure there has been no inadvertent mucosal perforation. An intra-operative photo of the pyloric tumour which has been incised can be seen in Figure 6.4.

Oral feeds may be commenced following a successful operation babies almost immediately following surgery, although some surgeons prefer to wait until the following morning before commencing feeds. rapidly regain their lost weight. The major complications of pyloromyotomy include mucosal perforation, wound infection, incisional hernia, prolonged postoperative emesis, incomplete myotomy and duodenal injury.

The key points in the management of IHPS are summarised next:

- A vomiting infant is not an unusual clinical situation.
- Resuscitation and appropriate fluid management is the essential first step prior to confirming the diagnosis.
- IV access should be achieved and bloods should be taken to determine the pH.
- It is usual to see a metabolic alkalosis with a paradoxical aciduria.
- USS is often equivocal in the early stages of disease and may need to be repeated.
- The placement of an NGT for gastric decompression and to allow for a thorough clinical examination for a pyloric tumour is necessary prior to aeromedical transfer.
- **Surgery is never scheduled until the acid-base imbalance has been corrected because of the significant risks of postoperative apnoeas in patients with uncorrected or partially corrected alkalosis.**

ANKYLOGLOSSIA

Ankyloglossia, also known as tongue-tie, is a short lingual frenum that interferes with normal tongue movement. The frequency seems to be higher in males, with a male-to-female ratio of 3:1. There is no standard definition of ankyloglossia. When examined, the "free tongue" length in newborns should be greater than 16 mm. Measurements of less than 11 mm indicate moderate ankyloglossia and less than 7 mm indicate severe ankyloglossia. Posterior ankyloglossia is used when the frenulum is attached in the middle to the posterior aspect of the undersurface of the tongue. In a minority of cases, the tongue-tie may sufficiently impair neonatal breastfeeding due to difficulty latching and consequently causing maternal discomfort and poor neonatal weight gain. In this specific subset of patients, surgical tongue-tie division is likely to improve breastfeeding. In the neonate, tongue-ties can be safely divided with or without general anaesthesia.

VASCULAR ANOMALIES IN CHILDREN

Abnormalities of either the blood vessels or lymphatic system are common in childhood. They may be evident at birth, or soon after, and are the cause of significant concern for most parents. There are many different types of vascular anomalies, which are generally classified according to the types of blood vessels involved. The cause of most of these anomalies is poorly understood and they may arise as part of a syndrome. The majority of these lesions are not detected antenatally and are small and do not cause clinical problems requiring surgery. The commonest vascular anomalies seen in everyday practice in children are haemangiomas.

Haemangiomas in Children

Haemangiomas are broadly classified as infantile (common) or congenital (rare). Infantile haemangiomas (IHs) are typically not present or are very small at birth and subsequently grow during infancy. In contrast, congenital haemangiomas (CHs) are fully developed at birth. Infantile haemangiomas have a characteristic growth pattern consisting of a rapid proliferative phase from 4 to 6 weeks of age and lasting for between 6 and 12 months. After this time, the IH usually plateaus in growth and is typically followed by a much slower involutional phase resulting in spontaneous resolution of >90% of IH by the age of 10 years. It is important to recognise those patients in whom more urgent surgical assessment is required. In particular, those patients with IH which may interfere with vision require urgent assessment as visual loss can be permanent. In children where IH is particularly disfiguring or in a position likely to cause problems, oral beta-blocker administration has been demonstrated to be highly effective medical treatment. It is important that patients are admitted and monitored carefully by the local paediatric team during initiation of treatment due to the potential for cardiac complications. Infantile haemangiomas are the only vascular tumour that respond to propranolol.

In contrast, CHs are far less common. They are often more purple in colour than the classic strawberry naevi (IH) and there is often an overlying telangiectasia. Within this group, there are three distinct variants:

- Rapidly involuting congenital haemangioma (RICH)
- Partially involuting congenital hemangioma (PICH)
- Non-involuting congenital haemangioma (NICH)

RICHs usually resolve completely within the first 6 months of life but can be life-threatening during the first few weeks of life due to AV shunting and cardiac failure. Very large lesions may require urgent surgery or embolisation. They may be associated with thrombocytopaenia due to platelet damage or consumption in the large vascular bed. This is often mistaken for Kasabach–Merritt phenomenon. The thrombocytopaenia is corrected as the tumour shrinks, but platelet transfusion can often increase consumption and cause the tumour to swell.

NICHs are often much smaller and usually asymptomatic.

PICHs represent a smaller subset of CHs which demonstrate features intermediate of RICHs and NICHs.

It is important to distinguish these singular lesions from patients with disseminated haemangiomatosis. Any patient with multiple skin lesions should be referred to a specialist vascular anomalies clinic for urgent assessment as they may have numerous liver lesions which can lead to abdominal compartment syndrome, cardiac failure and impaired liver function. They usually respond to treatment with propranolol.

Very rarely CHs may be part of a more extensive cluster of abnormalities (PHACE).

Two rarer vascular tumours can occur in childhood: Tufted angiomas and kaposiform haemangioendotheliomas. These are noteworthy as they are associated with Kasabach–Merritt phenomenon where profound thrombocytopaenia and low fibrinogen lead to potentially life-threatening bleeding. They may respond to treatment with sirolimus.

VASCULAR MALFORMATIONS

Vascular malformations are true congenital lesions in that they are present from birth although they may not be clinically evident until later. They are subdivided into low-flow (more common) and high-flow malformations. These malformations are usually managed by specialist clinics with the advice of surgeons, physicians (dermatologists and geneticists as well as paediatricians and oncologists) and interventional radiologists. Contemporary practice relies heavily on a multidisciplinary approach as diagnosis and treatment can be difficult. Management options include interventional radiology as well as specialist surgeons. Allied health is also useful in managing functional issues.

Venous Malformations

The most common form of low-flow vascular anomalies is venous malformation (VM). They have a complex classification beyond the scope of this chapter. In many instances, VMs are asymptomatic but they can cause pain and cosmetic issues. They may become more symptomatic during periods of rapid growth. Management strategies for VM are outlined next:

- Compression garments
- Sclerotherapy
- Surgery
- Cryoablation

Lymphatic Malformations

Lymphatic malformations arise due to congenital abnormalities of the lymphatic system resulting in a collection of thin-walled cysts containing lymphatic fluid. They can be diagnosed antenatally in some cases (e.g. cystic hygroma) or may become larger during intercurrent viral illnesses. Indications for treatment include mass effect, recurrent infections or functional issues. They are either microcystic or macrocystic in nature and macrocystic disease is usually effectively managed by percutaneous sclerotherapy after cyst drainage. Microcystic disease is much more difficult to treat effectively although bulk reduction with bleomycin treatment under US guidance may be effective.

Arteriovenous Malformations

Arteriovenous malformations (AVMs) are fast-flow vascular malformations characterised by abnormal connections or shunts between feeding arteries and draining veins without an intervening capillary bed. It is relatively rare for them to cause problems during childhood. Shunts are the nidus of the malformation. CNS AVMs are more common than extracranial AVMs. The purposes of the following discussion will be based upon extracranial AVMs. The fast flow through the shunt becomes more evident in childhood and adolescence as the lesion expands and develops into a mass. The overall risk of haemorrhage from an untreated AVM in all age groups is estimated to be between 2% and 4% yearly.

Pathogenesis

The direct AV shunting due to the lack of capillaries between the feeding arterial and draining venous components leads to hypertrophy in the arterial and venous components. The embryological basis of AVMs is due to either the persistence of a primitive AV connection or the development of a new connection after a normal closure process. It is hypothesised that most malformations occur during the third week of embryogenesis.

Clinical Presentation

On examination, lesions will palpate warm, with bruit or thrill. Puberty, pregnancy or local trauma tends to trigger more rapid expansion. Continued expansion leads to local tissue ischaemia and pain, therefore prompting treatment. The Schobinger clinical staging system for AVMs is mentioned in Table 6.1.

TABLE 6.1 The Schobinger clinical staging system for AVMs

STAGE	CLINICAL FEATURES
I (Quiescence)	Pink-bluish appearance, warmth and arteriovascular shunting demonstrated on Doppler USS
II (Expansion)	Same as Stage I plus enlargement, pulsations, thrills and bruit. Tortuous/tense veins may be visible
III (Destruction)	Same as Stage II plus either dystrophic skin changes, ulceration, bleeding, persistent pain or tissue necrosis
IV (Decompensation)	Same features as Stage III plus cardiac failure

Imaging

US and Doppler imaging can elucidate the fast flow of these lesions and distinguish them from venous malformation. On CT, dilated feeding arteries and veins are areas of contrast enhancement. MRI and MRA are the most useful modalities to demonstrate the full extent of lesions.

Treatment

The mainstays of treatment are angiographic embolisation alone or in combination with excision. Local recurrence following early intervention can complicate future procedures. Very well-localised stage I AVMs may be amenable to excision. Treatment during infancy is indicated in cases of heart failure. Embolisation should be directed to the nidus itself and the arteriovenous fistulae.

The preferred treatment strategy for an AVM typically consists of resection carried out 2–3 days following preoperative embolisation of the nidus. Angiographic embolisation facilitates the operation by decreasing bleeding. The goal of treatment should be complete excision of the lesion, including the nidus of the AVM and the involved skin. Unfortunately, some AVMs are extensive and often not amenable to an operative approach in which embolisation is used for palliation. For difficult AVMs of the extremities, amputation may be considered for distal lesions.

SKIN ABSCESSES AND KERION

Skin infections are a cause of significant morbidity in tropical paediatric populations. Management of skin infections need to take into consideration likely causative agent, severity of infection, natural progression of disease, treatment risks and side effects as well as patient factors.

The most common bacterial skin infections are caused by *Staphylococcus aureus* or *Streptococcus pyogenes*. Infections may present as impetigo, folliculitis or cellulitis. In the case of abscess formation, source control should be achieved through an incision and drainage. As an adjunct to incision and drainage, appropriate antibiotics should also be utilised. For gram-positive organisms such as those aforementioned, a penicillin agent is preferred. However, in tropical regions such as in far North Queensland, about 16% of staphylococcal infections are attributed to community-acquired methicillin-resistant *S. aureus* (MRSA) which requires treatment with alternative antibiotic classes such as vancomycin and clindamycin.

Burkholderia pseudomallei, the cause of melioidosis, is endemic in Northern Australia and Southeast Asia. The clinical manifestations of melioidosis range from localised infection to overwhelming sepsis and death. The most common manifestation is pneumonia, skin and soft-tissue infection, comprising 13%–24% of clinical presentations. Cutaneous melioidosis may be primary (presenting symptom is skin infection) or secondary (melioidosis at other sites in the body with incidental skin involvement). Cutaneous melioidosis can present as an ulcer (the most common presentation), pustule or as crusted erythematous lesions. Most primary cutaneous melioidosis cases present as a single lesion.

Fungal infections tend to thrive in tropical regions. A kerion is an abscess caused by fungal infection. It most often occurs on the scalp (tinea capitis), but it may also arise on any site exposed to the fungus such as face (tinea faciei) and upper limbs (tinea corporis). It presents as a boggy lump, several centimetres in diameter. If on the scalp, the kerion has localised alopecia around the vicinity. Regional lymphadenopathy and systemic infective symptoms may arise. Kerion is caused by dramatic immune response to a dermatophyte fungal infection. Diagnosis is based upon the characteristic appearance of a kerion. To confirm diagnosis, scrapings and hair samples may be taken from the affected area for microscopy and fungal culture. Secondary bacterial infection is common. Kerion should be treated by oral antifungal agents.

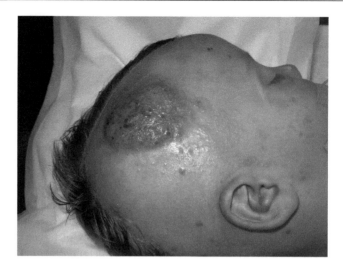

FIGURE 6.5   Kerion on scalp.

A course of 6–8 weeks of treatment is prescribed with interval clinical assessment. Kerions are commonly confused with abscesses or carbuncles and therefore are drained or excised, which can result in unnecessary scarring and ineffectual treatment. An example of a typical kerion can be seen in Figure 6.5.

Key Points

- Skin lesions are common in the tropics.
- Although abscesses are common when a boggy lump is seen on the scalp, the diagnosis of kerion should be considered.
- Treatment with incision and drainage of a kerion often results in a wound that is difficult to manage and takes a long time to heal.

SUMMARY

Infants commonly present to paediatric surgery department with a wide variety of different problems. It is important to recognise and to be able to treat the commonly occurring conditions. In particular, abscesses and skin lesions often cause a great deal of confusion and concern among parents. It is important to recognise those rarer cases that require urgent specialist attention to avoid unnecessary complications.

Conditions such as intussusception are frequently considered a diagnosis and it is important to proceed to resuscitation prior to trying to secure a definitive diagnosis; unfortunately many children have undergone marked deterioration in radiology departments whilst undergoing scans. It is important to ensure that clinicians anticipate and prepare for such eventualities.

The management of pyloric stenosis has moved from being an operation performed by general surgeons to one exclusively performed by paediatric surgeons in developed countries over the last 20 years. This has resulted in much improved outcomes for patients. The key to successful surgery lies in adequate preoperative resuscitation and utilisation of skilled paediatric anaesthetists for safe administration of general anaesthesia.

FURTHER READING

Cares K, El-Baba M. Rectal prolapse in children: Significance and management. Curr Gastroenterol Rep. 2016 May;18(5):22.

Gluckman S, Karpelowsky J, Webster AC, McGee RG. Management for intussusception in children. Cochrane Database Syst Rev. 2017 June;6(6):CD006476.

John AM, Schwartz RA, Janniger CK. The kerion: An angry tinea capitis. Int J Dermatol. 2018 January;57(1):3–9.

Kelley-Quon LI, et al. Management of intussusception in children: A systematic review. J Pediatr Surg. 2021 March;56(3):587–96.

O'Shea JE, Foster JP, O'Donnell CP, Breathnach D, Jacobs SE, Todd DA, Davis PG. Frenotomy for tongue-tie in newborn infants. Cochrane Database Syst Rev. 2017 March;3(3):CD011065.

Wassef M, et al. ISSVA Board and Scientific Committee. Vascular anomalies classification: Recommendations from the International Society for the Study of Vascular Anomalies. Pediatrics. 2015 July;136(1):e203–e14.

General Surgery in Childhood

7

Phoebe Leung, Harry Stalewski and Daniel Carroll

INTRODUCTION

It is common for children to present with surgical conditions in childhood. Roughly, one in ten children undergo surgery, a much larger number present either as emergencies or to outpatients for surgical problems; until recently, the majority of these children were not operated upon by specialist paediatric surgeons. Whilst not seeking to elaborate on areas covered in other chapters, it is important to possess a working knowledge of the surgical problems that present commonly in childhood. This is particularly relevant to practice in remote and rural settings where an understanding of these problems is particularly useful to allow appropriate recognition and timely referral of problems requiring specialist intervention. In such settings, these conditions are often managed by general surgeons and remote and regional medical specialists rather than specialist paediatric surgeons; it is useful to remember that one of the founding principles of the British Association of Paediatric Surgeons was 'to set a standard, not create a monopoly', and this sentiment is as relevant to practice today as it was in 1953; this is particularly true in our practice where patients and resources are spread over a large geographical area.

PRESENTATION

For the purposes of this chapter it is convenient to divide patients into different groups, as an understanding of the common presenting features of each condition is often helpful in establishing the correct diagnosis. Surgical problems often present as emergencies and in an unplanned fashion. The symptoms are often acute in onset, distressing for children and lead parents to seek medical attention promptly.

THE CHILD WITH ABDOMINAL PAIN

Patients presenting with abdominal pain make up a significant number of attendances to see both family doctors and emergency departments. Abdominal pain accounts for 5–10% of all presentations to paediatric emergency departments.

DOI: 10.1201/9781003156659-7

Assessment of the Child with Acute Abdominal Pain

The first and most important component in the successful management of a child with abdominal pain is to take a careful, and where necessary, detailed history from the child and the parents. Acute abdominal pain is defined as a pain of non-traumatic origin with a maximum duration of 5 days. While most emergency visits presenting with acute abdominal pain are self-limiting a surgical cause may be found in up to 20%, it is important to consider that in younger children, the incidence of surgical pathologies decreases, and paediatric medical diagnoses are much more common. In infants (children under the age of 1 year), the two most common surgical diagnoses are incarcerated inguinal hernia and ileocolic intussusception. These two conditions account for 90% of surgical cases in children under 1 year of age presenting as emergencies with acute abdominal pain.

In children under over 1 year of age, the most common surgical diagnosis is acute appendicitis (which accounts for roughly 2/3 of cases ultimately requiring surgery). The other common causes requiring surgery are incarcerated hernias, trauma and ileocolic intussusception. In contrast to what is seen in adults, the majority of children (2/3) present with suppurative or gangrenous appendicitis. It is often possible after taking a history and after a careful examination to establish a non-surgical cause of abdominal pain.

Acute Abdominal Pain in Children

It can be seen from Table 7.1 that the majority of conditions requiring surgery would not only be expected to manifest as abdominal pain, but also that, in general, the nature of that pain would be severe, not self-limiting, often becoming progressively worse and would be associated with abdominal tenderness and in particular guarding. These cardinal features of surgical causes of abdominal pain should lead to prompt assessment and referral to surgeon. Of particular significance to paediatric surgeons is the sign of bile-stained vomiting. Dark-green vomit is of particular concern to surgeons as it can be the only sign of intestinal obstruction – and of particular concern, a small bowel volvulus secondary to malrotation which requires urgent emergency surgery. Patients often present with more nebulous signs and symptoms, and in such cases, it is important to consider medical causes of abdominal pain, as failure to adequately treat and identify these problems (particularly sepsis) can lead to poor outcomes for children.

TABLE 7.1   Common causes of abdominal pain in children

Surgical	• Acute appendicitis
	• Ileocolic intussusception
	• Incarcerated inguinal hernia
	• Torsion of the testis
	• Meckel's diverticulum
	• Pancreatitis
	• Trauma
	• Psoas abscess
Medical	• Non-specific abdominal pain
	• Mesenteric adenitis
	• Gastroenteritis
	• Urosepsis
	• Hepatitis
	• Psychological
	• Non-accidental injury/child abuse/neglect
	• Lower lobe pneumonia
	• Henoch–Schonlein purpura
	• Diabetic ketoacidosis
Other	• Gynaecological
	• Musculoskeletal e.g. osteomyelitis, referred pain from hip

The Infant with Abdominal Pain

It is uncommon for children under 12 months of age present with surgical problems. The history is presumptive and often difficult, and the diagnosis of abdominal pain is often made on the basis of distress and crying. The pain is often described as colicky and may be associated with intermittent drawing up of the legs and settling between episodes of pain. It is important to recognise surgical causes as if they go unrecognised and untreated, there can be rapid clinical deterioration. The specific features that point to a surgical pathology are:

- Bile-stained vomiting
- The passage of blood per rectum
- Abdominal tenderness
- The presence of tender swellings in the abdomen or groin

Children THAT are critically unwell upon presentation require empiric resuscitation with fluids and antibiotics concomitant to the establishment of a definitive diagnosis.

ACUTE APPENDICITIS

Acute appendicitis is the most common surgical cause of patients presenting with acute abdominal pain. Around 3–5% of children undergo appendectomy during childhood, and the most common age of presentation is between the ages of 10 and 17 years. Reported mortality in higher income countries is low, but morbidity is higher in children than adults, with perforated or complicated appendicitis occurring in around 1:3 children. The risk of complicated appendicitis is higher in younger children, and perforated appendicitis is very common in patients under 5 years of age.

Clinical Features of Appendicitis

The common presenting features are of malaise and decrease appetite with associated abdominal pain and often vomiting. Classically, the pain is characterised as intermittent and periumbilical in nature initially with a subsequent localisation to the right lower quadrant. Unfortunately, younger children are often unreliable historians; however, the careful elucidation of a history of the nature of the pain is the cornerstone of making the correct diagnosis. When asked about symptoms, families will often volunteer that the child has had a fever with nausea and a loss of appetite (although anorexia is not universal, particularly in teenage boys!). By the time of presentation to hospital, there is often pain on movement, with an abnormal gait, which is exacerbated by sudden movements or bumps in the road during transfer. The vital signs that support acute appendicitis are a low-grade fever and a mild tachycardia.

Although the common features of appendicitis are widely known, only around 50% of children present with these classical features. If the diagnosis is delayed beyond 48 h (which is often the case in remote and rural communities), the perforation rate is around 2/3. After perforation, the localising signs are often less obvious, and the child may present with sepsis or obstructive symptoms.

Investigations

In general, clinical diagnosis is more accurate than the most widely performed investigations. In cases in which there is diagnostic uncertainty then a number of tests can be helpful, but often, repeated clinical examination is a better option.

A leucocytosis may occur as appendicitis worsens, but is often normal in early appendicitis. Urinalysis is commonly performed in children as urinary tract infections are a common cause of abdominal pain. Often in appendicitis the urinalysis is normal, but around 25% of patients have white cells or red cells present in their urine at the time of presentation, and so it is important to also look for bacteria in a clean catch urine specimen with formal urine microscopy and culture.

Around 50% of patients can be diagnosed clinically without the need for further investigations.

Radiological investigations

Ultrasound scanning (USS) is widely used in the assessment of children with acute abdominal pain. It has the advantage of being widely available, even in remote and rural settings, it is relatively cheap and has been reported as high levels of sensitivity (80–85%) and specificity (90–95%) when diagnosing appendicitis. It is important to note that the majority of these studies have been performed by skilled operators in children's hospitals, and it is unlikely that such high levels of sensitivity and specificity can be replicated in the hands of those less accustomed to performing USS examinations in children on a regular basis. The ultrasonographic features suggestive of appendicitis include probe tenderness over the appendix, a transverse diameter of the appendix greater than 6 mm and a non-compressible appendix. Ultrasound is most useful in looking for ovarian pathology in post-pubertal females, as it is important to rule this out prior to planning for surgery. It is important to remember to only use supporting investigations when clinical diagnosis alone is not able to come to a satisfactory conclusion.

CT scanning is more accurate than USS with reported sensitivity and specificity of around 95%. It can be of particular value in obese children but is not commonly used due to the long-term risks of cancer development as a consequence of radiation exposure. It very rarely is indicated. Paediatric surgeons have been repeatedly demonstrated to be about 95% accurate in diagnosing appendicitis using selective observation, repeated clinical examination and selected blood tests. The use of poorly timed and indiscriminate investigations increases costs, causes diagnostic confusion and delay and should be avoided.

Treatment of Appendicitis

The treatment of non-complicated appendicitis consists of:

- Preoperative resuscitation as required
- The administration of appropriate analgesia (including opiates)
- Early institution of antibiotics after coming to a definitive clinical diagnosis
- Appendectomy (discussed later in this book)

There is currently insufficient data to support conservative treatment of appendicitis in children. Although this is becoming more common in the adult population, early data suggests that recidivism with further episodes of appendicitis is more common in the paediatric population.

In the case of complicated appendicitis (generalised peritonitis supporting a diagnosis of perforation), surgical exploration and aggressive irrigation should be performed, once the patient has been adequately resuscitated as in the treatment of simple appendicitis. For those patients with signs of shock or intestinal obstruction, the placement of a urinary catheter to monitor urine output, routine bloods and the placement of a nasogastric tube to decompress the stomach should all be considered. These measures are particularly important in remote settings where there may be considerable delay in transferring patients to a tertiary level facility and the use of aeromedical retrieval means intestinal decompression is necessary.

In rare cases of perforated appendicitis with subsequent appendix mass formation treatment should initially be supportive and conservative rather than surgical. Physiological support (including adequate pain relief and nutrition) and intravenous antibiotics guided by local antimicrobial policies are often successful, although the data suggests that subsequent interval appendectomy is probably indicated. This is particularly true in patients coming from remote areas.

THE ACUTE SCROTUM

Presentation to the emergency department because of concerns about acute pain in the testis is common in children. The acute scrotum is defined as the constellation of sudden onset of pain and or tenderness or swelling and redness in the scrotum or its contents. It is important to expeditiously assess children to determine the cause of the pain, as testicular torsion must be considered in any patient who complains of acute scrotal pain and swelling.

Testicular Torsion

Torsion of the testis is a surgical emergency as the likelihood of testicular salvage decreases as the duration of torsion increases. The initiation of investigations should never delay the prompt referral to the relevant surgical team to prevent unnecessary testicular loss. Whilst it is important not to delay treatment, certain features both in the clinical history and signs found on physical examination can help differentiate between the different causes of acute testicular pain. A number of conditions can mimic testicular torsion, most commonly a torsion of a testicular appendage (particularly in prepubertal boys) and less commonly in children epididymo-orchitis, trauma, hernia, hydrocoele, Henoch–Schonlein purpura (HSP) and idiopathic scrotal oedema (ISE).

The following signs and symptoms are the cardinal features of testicular torsion:

• Acute onset of severe pain
• Vomiting/anorexia/nausea
• Testicular tenderness
• A horizontal testicular lie
• Abolition of the cremasteric reflex

It is quite possible for none of these features to be present and to still find a torsion of the testis at surgical exploration. In regional and rural practice, and, in particular, in remote tropical areas, practical considerations often mean that patients cannot undergo immediate scrotal exploration. In such cases, urinalysis and Doppler USS examination of the scrotum may have a limited role in allowing the relative likelihood of a genuine testicular torsion to be present when immediate surgical exploration is not available. There is unfortunately considerable overlap in the clinical features of acute testicular torsion and torsion of a testicular or epididymal appendage. It is the author's practice to urgently explore almost all boys with testicular tenderness. The clinical features of the common causes of the scrotum are listed below (Table 7.2).

TABLE 7.2   Common causes of the acute scrotum

CONDITION	ONSET	AGE	TENDERNESS	URINALYSIS
		FEATURES OF COMMON CAUSES OF THE ACUTE SCROTUM		
Testicular torsion	Acute	Post-pubertal	Diffuse and cord	–
Epidiymo-orchitis	Insidious	Post-pubertal	Epididymal	+/– leuc
Appendix torsion	Subacute	Prepubertal	Discrete area	–
HSP	Subacute	Prepubertal	Diffuse	+/– rbc
Idiopathic SE	Subacute	Prepubertal	None	–

Torsion of Testicular Appendages

The appendix testis is a Mullerian duct remnant located at the superior pole of the testis. It is the most common appendage to undergo torsion; the epididymal appendage (a Wolffian duct remnant) may also become twisted. Torsion of either appendage produces pain and tenderness similar to that seen in a true testicular torsion; patients are usually prepubertal in age, and the onset and severity of the pain is often less than that seen in acute testicular torsion. Unfortunately, USS is not sufficiently specific as a test to completely exclude testicular torsion. On occasion, a 'blue dot' may be visible through the scrotal skin, particularly if patients present early prior to the development of scrotal oedema of the overlying skin, this allows a clinical diagnosis of a torsion of a testicular appendage to be made with reasonable certainty, and it is possible to offer the family a conservative approach to management. This is particularly useful in remote practice as it may avoid the need for urgent exploration and transfer of the patient. Boys with this condition can sometimes experience ongoing debilitating pain and worsening of symptoms even with simple analgesia, and a conservative strategy may be unsuccessful in such cases. In prepubertal males, the incidence of torsion of the testicular or epididymal appendage is significantly more common than a genuine torsion of the testis.

Epididymo-Orchitis

Epididymo-orchitis is uncommon in prepubertal males. It has long been recommended that urinalysis is performed in males with an acute scrotum to try and identify patients with epididymo-orchitis and thus avoid unnecessary urgent scrotal exploration. However, urinalysis may be negative even in the presence of bacterial epididymo-orchitis. Urine microscopy, culture and sensitivities can be helpful in guiding subsequent antimicrobial therapy if epididymo-orchitis is suspected. Any episode of epididymo-orchitis in childhood should be investigated with renal tract ultrasonography to look for structural renal tract abnormalities. Treatment is with antibiotics; it is not uncommon for patients to require an extended course of antibiotics to successfully treat bacterial epididymo-orchitis, and usually, we recommend a course of 2 weeks ciprofloxacin in the first instance. The majority of cases in younger patients are viral in nature, but it is difficult to exclude bacterial infections as urinalysis is often normal. Patients with recurrent epididymo-orchitis may be due to abnormalities in the proximal urethra such as an enlarged prostatic utricle with abnormal vasal reflux, such patients may require further investigations such as cystoscopy to investigate for possible anatomical abnormalities.

Scrotal Trauma

Severe testicular injury is fortunately uncommon in childhood, but a direct blow to the scrotum or a straddle injury can result in an intratesticular haematoma or laceration of the tunica albuginea. Such cases require immediate drainage and repair. Traumatic epididymitis is one potential sequela of scrotal trauma, and a conservative strategy may be adopted if there are no concerns about damage to the tunica albuginea. Ultrasonography in skilled hands can be useful in such cases.

Henoch–Schonlein Purpura (HSP)

HSP is a systemic vasculitic syndrome. It is characterised by a non-thrombocytopenic purpura. This can cause a variety of symptoms, including arthralgia, renal disease (manifesting as a microscopic haematuria on urinalysis and microscopy), abdominal pain and gastrointestinal bleeding. Classically, a purpuric rash is often noticed on the shins. HSP occasionally presents as acute testicular pain, and if there are other supporting features or the diagnosis is suspected, then they should be assessed by a paediatrician as well.

Idiopathic Scrotal (O)Edema (ISE)

Acute idiopathic scrotal oedema (ISE) is another possible cause of an acute scrotum. The aetiology of this condition is unclear, but the patient presents with a red or swollen scrotum. Classically, the oedema and redness are described as bilateral and symmetrical; however, it is the author's experience that often it can start on one side and then spread across the median raphe over time. Although the appearance of the scrotum may be quite florid and certainly alarming to the parents and clinicians, the cardinal feature of this condition is a distinct lack of tenderness of either testis or the cord. The cremasteric reflex is usually maintained. Treatment is with bed rest/elevation/analgesia (although pain is often not a clinical feature). There is some evidence that antihistamines may reduce the duration of clinical features. (An example of a male infant with ISE can be seen in Figure 7.1.)

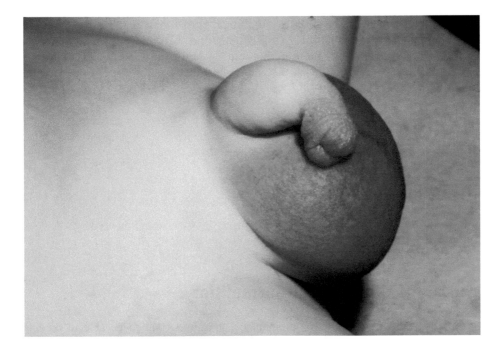

FIGURE 7.1 Idiopathic scrotal oedema.

Inguinal hernia/Hydrocoeles

Occasionally, obstructed or incarcerated inguinal hernia can manifest as an acute scrotum. A fuller description of the management of these conditions can be found in Chapter 6.

UMBILICAL HERNIA

It is a very common occurrence to find an umbilical abnormality at birth, particularly in premature infants. The estimated incidence of umbilical hernia in neonates is between 20 and 30% at birth, and the incidence is higher in premature infants with a reported incidence of 85% in children with a birth weight between 1000 and 1500 g. The incidence is higher in some ethnic groups; it is also more commonly seen in patients with a variety of other medical conditions, including trisomy 21, mucopolysaccharidoses and other congenital abnormalities.

The commonest umbilical abnormality at birth is an umbilical hernia; the vast majority of these will close spontaneously by the age of 4–5 years (over 90%). It is important to understand the aetiology and embryology, as well as to be able to recognise other umbilical pathologies to allow for appropriate advice and information to be given to families and to ensure that patients are referred appropriately to paediatric surgical services.

Embryology and Anatomy

During early fetal development, the primitive umbilical ring forms on the ventral surface of the fetus between the 4th and 5th weeks of fetal life. The primitive umbilical ring contains a number of structures: the umbilical vessels (two arteries and one vein), the vitelline duct and vessels and the allantois as well as a loop of midgut. The herniated midgut returns to the abdomen and, in doing so, leads to the development of the definitive umbilical cord which contains the umbilical vessels encased in Wharton's jelly. The umbilical vessels obliterate soon after birth and are replaced with a ligamentous structure. Failure of these normal embryological processes can result in a number of congenital disorders of the umbilicus, the commonest being umbilical hernia. The commonest abnormalities are:

- Umbilical hernia
- Patent urachus
- Omphalomesenteric fistula
- Umbilical polyp
- Umbilical granuloma
- Hernia of the cord

Assessment of Umbilical Abnormalities

Although umbilical abnormalities are commonplace, it is important to be able to recognise other umbilical problems as they may require more specialised assessment and intervention. Any abnormal finding in a neonate should prompt a more detailed evaluation of the infant, including the taking of an antenatal and family history. Umbilical hernia is more common in a number of important conditions, including:

- Trisomy 21 and 18 and other chromosomal abnormalities
- Beckwith–Wiedemann syndrome
- Marfan's syndrome
- Hypothyroidism
- Mucopolysaccharidoses

It is important to look for other stigmata of these conditions and to examine the umbilical region carefully. It is important to look at the size of the defect; typically, very large defects (2–3 cm) are uncommon but are less likely to close spontaneously; it is important to distinguish between the size of the defect in the fascia rather than the size of the skin defect, which can often be large even with relatively small defect. It is important to examine the umbilicus carefully to look for persistent discharges or ectopic mucosae which are signs of a patent urachus or persistent vitellointestinal duct remnant. These abnormalities require further assessment by a paediatric surgeon.

Management of Umbilical Abnormalities

Surgical repair of umbilical defects is usually deferred until children are between 2 and 5 years of age. The risk of complications due to incarceration of intestinal contents is low in childhood. It is possible for intestinal contents or omentum to become incarcerated and require emergent surgical treatment, but this is uncommon with an incidence of around 1:10,000 cases per year. Many parents are concerned about the size of the swelling, particularly if the hernia is large and protuberant, although these herniae are less likely to become incarcerated or obstructed. A number of attempts have been made to strap or tape umbilical herniae to encourage them to close, but unfortunately, these techniques have been of little demonstrable value and are associated with an increase in the incidence of potential complications. In our practice in remote and regional areas, it is often practical to repair uncomplicated umbilical herniae in children towards the younger end of the age range to prevent unnecessary parental anxiety as patients often live significant distances from a paediatric surgeon. (An example of an infant with a large umbilical hernia can be seen in Figure 7.2.)

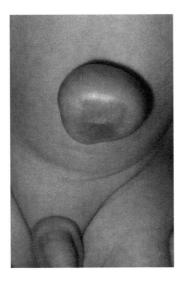

FIGURE 7.2   Umbilical hernia.

Emergency surgery is indicated for complications of the hernia, which are fortunately uncommon. Occasionally, an umbilical hernia may become incarcerated (often with omentum present in a smaller defect), and there are reports of intestinal strangulation and obstruction and even of rupture secondary to trauma. In children with larger fascial defects (>1.5 cm) that persist beyond 2 years of age, these rarely close spontaneously, and so repair is recommended. There is little value in deferring surgery in these patients as the risk of surgery is little changed between the age of 2 and 5 years.

Umbilical hernia repair is more correctly termed an umbilical herniotomy. An infra-umbilical incision is made, and then the hernial sac and defect are circumscribed. The hernia sac is then opened, and the fascial defect is closed with an absorbable suture. This can typically be performed as a day case surgery. It is uncommon to have to use mesh to facilitate a repair in children, but it may be necessary in very large defects (>5 cm); these are probably more correctly thought of as covered anterior abdominal wall defects. Umbilicoplasty may be performed for those patients particularly with large skin defects that are protuberant in nature.

Complications and Long-Term Management

Unfortunately, it is difficult to ascertain the true rate of complications in patients with untreated umbilical hernias as there is significant selection bias in the published data. From our experience, in those patients who have umbilical hernia but only have limited access to surgery (e.g. in developing countries) we know that complications of untreated umbilical hernias are rare in childhood. The reported incidence of complications in untreated umbilical hernias is between 1:300 and 1000. As children progress into adult life, the risk of complications becomes higher, particularly in pregnancy; the rationale behind fixing these hernias in childhood is to prevent these complications later, and the surgery is relatively safe and straightforward in younger children. Umbilical hernia repairs have a low postoperative complication rate. The commonest early complication is a superficial wound infection, prompting the use of routine perioperative antibiotics. After routine repair, recurrence is uncommon (1–2%) except in those patients with underlying predisposition to hernia formation (trisomy 21, mucopolysaccharidoses, connective tissue disorders). Longer-term follow-up is recommended for this selected group of patients.

ABNORMALITIES OF TESTICULAR DESCENT

Abnormalities of testicular descent are a common problem in everyday practice. A failure of the normal processes of testicular descent is termed *testicular maldescent*. This can be further classified as:

- Undescended testis
- Ectopic testis
- Ascending testis
- Retractile testis
- Absent testis

Perhaps most usefully testes can be divided up practically into two main groups, *palpable* (but abnormally positioned) and *impalpable*.

Undescended Testes

The second most common condition requiring paediatric surgery in childhood is testicular maldescent. The reported incidence varies according to the population being studied (e.g. age and other factors such

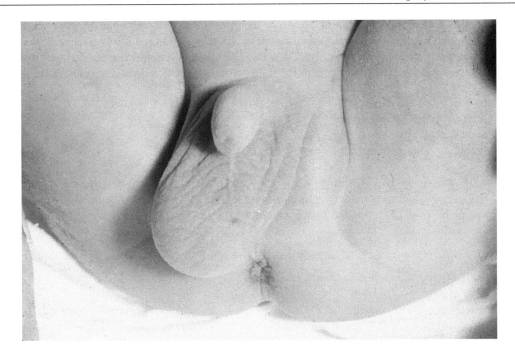

FIGURE 7.3   Empty left hemiscrotum (left undescended testis).

as prematurity), but a widely accepted figure is that around 1:60 boys undergo surgery for undescended testis in the first 2 years of life. An example of a child with an undescended testis with a clearly empty left hemiscrotum can be seen in Figure 7.3.

At birth, up to 10% of term infants are identified as having some abnormality of testicular descent. By the age of 3–6 months, this falls to around 2–3% of boys. It is important that these patients are followed up carefully, and that boys who are determined clinically to have testicular maldescent at 3 months of age or older are referred to a paediatric surgeon for assessment and ongoing management.

In the majority of cases, testicular descent is unilateral; however, it is important to acknowledge the increased clinical significance of boys with bilateral testicular maldescent; in such cases, examination of the external genitalia should be performed by a specialist to exclude disorders of sexual differentiation. In cases of bilateral impalpable testes, or in cases with other abnormalities of the external genitalia (e.g. hypospadias, bifid scrotum), urgent paediatric surgical/urological referral is warranted.

To fully understand the different forms of testicular maldescent, a basic understanding of the embryology and pathophysiology of normal testicular descent is required.

Normal Mechanisms of Testicular Descent

There are two independent stages of testicular descent; the first stage termed the *abdominal phase* occurs between 8 and 15 weeks of gestation. The gubernaculum tethers the developing gonad to the region of the internal ring resulting in its migration to the location in the developing male fetus during the second trimester. This phase is dependent upon anti-Mullerian hormone (AMH) and functioning AMH receptors but is independent of androgens and functional androgen receptors. If this first stage of testicular descent fails them, the testis remains intra-abdominal.

The second phase of testicular descent is more complex, and as such, more commonly goes awry. The second phase of testicular descent is termed the *inguinal phase*. After the testis has reached the internal ring, the gubernaculum continues to expand and extends into the scrotum. Under the influence of androgens, virilisation of the genitofemoral nerve results in the local production of calcitonin gene related peptide (CGRP) which is through to cause the gubernaculum to rhythmically contract, drawing the testis through the inguinal canal to its ultimate destination within the scrotum. It is clear that testicular maldescent can occur for a variety of different reasons as it is dependent upon complex series of sequential events. For successful descent of the testis into the scrotum to occur, we must have:

- A correctly sited gubernaculum
- Adequate fetal virilisation
- Normal hormonal balance during the third trimester

Emerging evidence suggests that disruptions in the normal fetal hormonal balance caused by disturbances in intrauterine hormonal function are important contributors to testicular maldescent. Commonly cited risks for testicular maldescent include:

- Family history of undescended testis
- Maternal history
- IUGR
- Prematurity
- Intrauterine exposure to high levels of oestrogen

However, the causal mechanisms behind these observations are yet to be established.

There is evidence that testes that fail to descend normally are intrinsically abnormal (both macroscopically and microscopically). Histological studies have demonstrated that dysplastic elements are commonly seen. These abnormalities in combination with the non-physiological temperature environment of the undescended testis are thought to contribute to the increased risk of malignant transformation of undescended testes. The temperature within the scrotum is around 3°C lower than body temperature. The complex nature of the mechanisms underpinning normal testicular descent into the scrotum results in the relatively common incidence of testicular maldescent.

Diagnosis

It is important to take every opportunity to examine the external genitalia of male infants when they come to see a doctor or healthcare professional. This is of particular importance in areas where healthcare resources are unevenly distributed such as remote practice. The first opportunity to do so is at the routine baby check. For the vast majority of male infants, it is relatively straightforward at this stage to palpate both testes in the scrotum, and it is usual for it to remain straightforward for the first few months of life. Once children are older, and the cremasteric reflex becomes more established in male infants over 6 months of age, the assessment of testicular position is more challenging. This is particularly true if the child is frightened, upset, cold or crying, and in such instances, parents will often be able to recall if they have seen the testes in the scrotum. Ideally, the physical examination should take place in an unhurried manner, in a warm room with a calm child. A well-developed hemiscrotum is usually a sign that a testis has at least at some point been within the scrotum. Conversely, an underdeveloped hemiscrotum suggests that the testis has not come to occupy a satisfactory scrotal position, as normal scrotal development and virilisation are dependent upon local production and tissue response to androgens by a testicle situated within the hemiscrotum. If the testis is palpable, then it may be mobile, but it is important to determine testicular volume and position and to recognise whether it can be drawn to the base of the scrotum and whether it reascends upon release.

Classification of Testicular Maldescent

If a testis is maldescended, it can be divided into two major categories, *palpable* (80%) or *impalpable* (20%). For palpable testes, these can then be classified according to their position in relation to the inguinal canal. Impalpable testes are either absent (50%), intra-abdominal (40%) or canalicular (10%). Most commonly undescended testes sit in the superficial inguinal pouch, whereas retractile testes occupy a high scrotal position but can be drawn into the hemiscrotum and remain there without tension upon release. When a testis has been documented as palpable and descended but comes to occupy a less satisfactory position as the child grows, this is termed the *ascending testis*, although the author prefers the term 'stationary testis' as it more precisely describes the fixed position of the testis in relation to the external ring.

Management of Testicular Maldescent

Current guidelines recommend referral between the ages of 3 and 6 months for boys with unilateral, uncomplicated testicular maldescent. Those with complicating features, such as bilateral impalpable testes or additional abnormalities of the external genitalia (such as hypospadias or bifid scrotum), should be referred urgently to paediatric surgical or paediatric urological services dependent upon local availability.

Patients with testicular maldescent should undergo corrective surgery as soon as is safe and practical. Some surgeons now advocate earlier surgery than previously recommended (between the ages of 3 and 6 months). Theoretically, this will improve long-term prospects for fertility and reduce the longer-term risk of carcinogenesis; however, most surgeons outside of large specialist centres aim to perform surgery around 9–12 months of age when the risk of complications and general anaesthesia are considered to be somewhat lower. In practice, it is important to refer patients as soon as is practical if testicular maldescent persists beyond 3 months of age to allow for timely surgery.

Investigations

USS is widely performed prior to referral; however, it is not usually useful. It has a low sensitivity (78%) and even lower specificity (45%) in determining testicular position and in locating an impalpable testis. In general, clinical examination is superior in determining the need for surgery and in deciding what surgery will be required.

Surgical Management

Testes that are palpable are usually relatively straightforward to deal with operatively. These patients should ideally undergo an open orchidopexy between 9 and 12 months of age. Through an inguinal incision, the testis is identified, and any hernia sac or fibrotic remains of the patent processus vaginalis are divided. This manoeuvre usually allows for the testis to be easily delivered to the base of the scrotum via a scrotal incision without tension. The testis is then placed in a subdartos pouch and secured to the median raphe with absorbable sutures. Closure of the scrotum is best performed with an absorbable suture such as chromic as it is my experience that rapidly absorbing sutures such as vicryl rapide absorb too quickly in the tropical environment. The success rate for an open orchidopexy is reported to be around 90–95%, although complications such as testicular atrophy and reascent do occur and should be openly discussed with the family as part of the consent process, particularly in patients with bilateral testicular maldescent.

Patients with impalpable gonads require a slightly more involved approach. Most surgeons choose to examine the child under anaesthesia and if the testis remains impalpable under these conditions proceed to laparoscopy to determine whether the testis is absent, intra-abdominal or canalicular. In the case of a solitary testis, it is my usual practice to fix the remaining testis because of the subsequent risk of testicular torsion. This is particularly pertinent in remote practice, as the chances of being able to get to hospital for scrotal exploration in a timely manner are significantly lower than for those patients living in metropolitan areas. If the testis is intra-abdominal, it is possible to a single-stage or more commonly a two-stage laparoscopic Fowler–Stephens procedure. In this operation, pioneered in Melbourne, the testicular vessels are divided and the testis freed and mobilised on the vas deferens (and it's attendant vessels), prior to subsequent laparoscopic or open placement into the scrotum. Very high success rates have been reported for the two-stage procedures, but I suspect the true rates of long-term testicular survival without reascent are in the range of 70–80%.

Prognosis

Parents are usually quite reasonably concerned about the outlook for fertility and the longer-term risk of testicular cancer in boys with testicular maldescent. As previously mentioned, histological studies of the undescended testis have demonstrated histological abnormalities in the undescended testis from a very early age. It is not uncommon during operation to demonstrate testicular and epididymal abnormalities (e.g. testiculo-epidiymal dislocation), and although the clinical significance of these findings has not been examined in any great detail, then it would seem likely that these will have some impact on sperm production or delivery into the ejaculate. A complete lack of germ cells has been reported in patients as young as 15 months, and there is some understandable concern that testes should be brought into the scrotum as soon as possible.

Despite these concerns, the outlook for fertility is quite good for boys with unilateral testicular maldescent. In larger studies, only small differences in sperm count have been demonstrated in men who have undergone unilateral orchidopexy and even smaller reported differences in self-reported paternity (89% compared to 94% in the normal population).

Unsurprisingly, for boys with bilateral testicular maldescent, the long-term results of surgery have been less encouraging. The infertility rate has been reported to be up to 50–60%, with associated significantly lower sperm density when compared to controls. Theoretically, early surgery may be of some benefit to this group, although currently, there is a paucity of long-term follow-up studies to support this.

The subsequent long-term risk of testicular cancer has been approximated as between 1 and 2% in patients with undescended testes. It is for this reason that it is essential to ensure a satisfactory scrotal position of the testis as soon as possible to allow young men to adequately perform routine testicular self-examination. Estimates as to the relative risks of malignancy lie between 5 and 10 compared to the background population, but this is dependent upon a number of other factors most notably testicular position at the time of operation with the highest risk being seen in those boys with late recognition and treatment of intra-abdominal testes.

Summary

- Testicular maldescent is common (1:30–60).
- Surgery is the only effective treatment currently for testicular maldescent.
- Subfertility is largely a concern for boys with bilateral testicular maldescent.
- The increased relative risk of malignancy requires long-term follow-up, and routine testicular self-examination should be encouraged.

NECK SWELLINGS

It is common for children to present with parental concerns regarding a lump in the neck. Whilst they are usually managed in primary care, by paediatricians or by ENT surgeons, it is not uncommon for children to be referred to paediatric surgeons for further investigation and management. In general, it is a helpful approach to divide masses up in relation to their position in the neck. Swellings may be midline or lateral and may increase rapidly in size or be present over a longer period of time. Careful history taking and physical examination often allow a differential diagnosis to be established prior to deciding the appropriate sequence of investigations. Some of the commoner lesions are listed in the following table:

CONGENITAL	INFECTIVE	NEOPLASTIC
Midline	Acute	Benign
Thyroglossal cyst	Reactive lymphadenopathy	Pilomatrixoma
Ectopic thyroid	Lymphadenitis	Lipomas
Dermoid cyst	Abscess	Neural tumours
Lateral	Chronic	Malignant
Branchial cleft/arch anomalies	Atypical/non-TB mycobacterial	Lymphoma
Torticollis	TB	Thyroid malignancies
SCM tumour	Toxoplasmosis/HIV	
	Goitre	
Other		
Haemangiomas		
Vascular: AVM/venous		
Lymphangioma		

Conditions of the Thyroid

Persistent thyroglossal duct and thyroglossal cysts

A persistent thyroglossal duct is one of the most common lesions in the midline of the neck and occurs in approximately 7% of the population. They generally present with symptoms typically seen in the pre-school age: 3–5 years old. An example of a child with an infected thyroglossal cyst can be seen in Figure 7.4.

Basic embryology

The thyroglossal duct is a congenital remnant which connects the posterior aspect of the tongue to the thyroid gland during embryological development. It originates from the foramen caecum which is where the thyroid diverticulum develops. At weeks 4–7, the thyroid migrates inferiorly from the foramen caecum past the base of the tongue and hyoid bone. The thyroid remains connected to the foramen caecum by the thyroglossal duct which is lined by lymphoid and epithelial cells. By the 3rd month, the duct typically disintegrates as the ductal walls adhere to itself and obliterate the canal.

Pathophysiology of thyroglossal duct remnants/cysts

In some children, the thyroglossal duct fails to involute completely. When mucus is secreted from the epithelial cells lining the duct, this subsequently prevents the adherence of the ductal walls. Collections of mucus in pockets within the duct allow cysts to form.

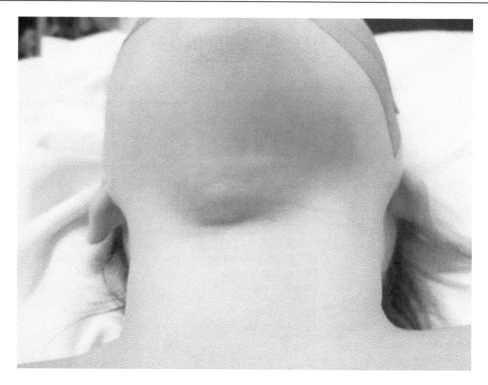

FIGURE 7.4   Infected thyoglossal cyst.

Clinical presentation

Overall, 75% of these occur near or attached to the hyoid bone, whilst others occur in the suprahyoid or subhyoid position. Children will typically present with a painless swelling in the midline of the anterior neck. This mass moves with swallowing or protrusion of the tongue due to the embryological attachment discussed earlier.

Due to its proximity and the presence of lymphoid cells, local inflammation stimulates mucus secretion and thus increases the size of the cyst. Other symptoms or complications include erythema and pain (33%), a discharging sinus (25%) or a foul taste depending on the patency of the duct. Erythema and pain are symptoms associated with an infected cyst. Thyroglossal cysts are usually diagnosed clinically but can be further evaluated with a US or CT scan if unclear.

Management of thyroglossal cyst

Primarily, the goal of treatment is to excise the entire tract – the Sistrunk procedure. But if it is infected, a course of antibiotics may be required prior to excision.

Ectopic thyroid tissue

Occasionally, cells of the thyroid gland can be found in the thyroglossal duct. This is concerning as it may indicate a hypoplastic thyroid and increases the risk of a thyroid tumour developing in the cyst. Early suspicion of an ectopic thyroid arises from abnormal thyroid function levels which are completed as part of the newborn screen. On palpation, they may be softer than a thyroglossal cyst but may only be discovered on excision. Radioisotopes can be used to determine if the ectopic thyroid is the only thyroid tissue present at which excision should not occur.

Dermoid and Epidermoid Cysts

Dermoid cysts can be difficult to delineate from thyroglossal cysts. Like thyroglossal cysts, they also present as midline masses which move with swallowing. However, dermoid cysts are typically more superficial and mobile. Most dermoid cysts are in the suprahyoid or submental area and filled with sebaceous material. During surgical excision, examination of the contents of the cyst may help differentiate the two pathologies.

Epidermoid cysts are lined with epidermis and do not contain sebaceous or mucous material. These can arise congenitally or are acquired due to traumatic entrapment of epidermis into the dermis/subcutaneous tissue. They are associated with sinus tracts and can be mistaken as branchial cleft remnants. The presence of multiple epidermoid cysts should raise the suspicion of Gardner's syndrome. Both dermoid and epidermoid cysts are excised due to their risk of rupture and infection which follows.

Thyroid Malignancies

Thyroid malignancies are rare in childhood. They usually come to the attention of medical professionals due to parental concerns about a new swelling appearing in the neck. Thyroid malignancies are more likely to present with cervical lymphadenopathy than a swelling due to a goitre. Risk factors include radiation exposure including CT scans and radiation treatment for other conditions. Overall, 90% of paediatric thyroid cancer comprises papillary thyroid cancer. Follicular thyroid malignancies are rare, whilst medullary carcinomas are frequently diagnosed in association with MEN syndrome. Hodgkin's lymphoma (HL) is the most common malignancy associated with secondary thyroid malignancies. The main causes of goitres include Hashimoto thyroiditis, Graves' disease, iodine deficiency or excessive maternal iodine intake during pregnancy.

BRANCHIAL CLEFT/ARCH ANOMALIES

Basic Embryology of Brachial Cleft Abnormalities

During week 3 of embryological development, gastrulation occurs, and the three pluripotent germ cell layers develop – the endoderm, mesoderm and ectoderm. Within the pharyngeal apparatus which forms the primitive pharynx, these three layers correlate to the pouch, cleft and arch. Initially, there are six branchial arches from the pharyngeal apparatus; however, the fifth typically regresses; thus, only five remain. Branchial cleft or arch anomalies usually develop from remnants of the first, second and third branchial systems.

The second branchial system is the most common pathology and starts in the tonsillar fossa. It then passes next to the glossopharyngeal nerve, between the internal and external carotids to the anterior border of the lower third of the sternocleidomastoid muscle (SCM).

The first branchial system anomalies manifest uncommonly, and its path begins at the external auditory canal and passes to the cutaneous surface below the inferior border of mandible.

Rarely, the third branchial system persists with the opening lying internally at the piriform sinus and traces to the cutaneous surface of the anterior border of the sternocleidomastoid.

Branchial arch anomalies present as atypical mesodermal remnants along the arch's development. The most common is the second branchial arch remnant which presents as a skin tag at the cutaneous opening. These are excised generally for cosmetic reasons.

Persisting branchial clefts (between arches) can form sinuses, fistulas or cysts. Branchial sinuses are the most common and are blind-ending canals with a cutaneous orifice whilst fistulas occur when there is a communication between two epithelial lined surfaces. They typically present with mucous leaking from the opening, or a recurrent wet spot noted on clothing. Tracts can occasionally be palpable and may excrete mucus when massaged.

Sinus and fistulas are usually lined by respiratory epithelium, whilst cysts are typically lined by squamous epithelium. Rarely, branchial cysts persist and are remnants of sinuses without a cutaneous orifice. All three pathologies are at risk of infection and require surgical complete excision to prevent recurrence. Depending on the clinical suspicion, further investigations including injection of radio-opaque liquid into the orifice, or a US/CT/MRI can be used to define the tract.

Sternocleidomastoid pathology

Congenital torticollis is a postural deformity commonly caused by the fibrosis of the SCM, causing shortening and the deviation of the neck *towards the side of the lesion*. It has been associated with a muscular injury sustained during a difficult birth or even prior to delivery. A suspicion of acquired torticollis should involve an investigation into ophthalmological (strabismus), otolaryngological (infection) or gastrointestinal pathology (gastro-oesophageal reflux disease [GORD]).

It is typically seen unilaterally but may occur bilaterally. Unilaterally, the infant has a classical appearance – ***the head is rotated away from the side of the lesion and with contralateral lateral flexion***. Most cases resolve with conservative management involving physiotherapy. Surgical intervention is considered when conservative management fails, for patients with a severe rotational deficit, or for those with prolonged symptoms.

Physical examination of a unilateral torticollis with a sternocleidomastoid mass is clinically suspicious of a sternocleidomastoid tumour. Key features include a 2–3 cm long hard, painless and spindle-shaped swelling in neonates 2–3 weeks old. It is commonly associated with plagiocephaly due to the impressionable skull and prolonged lying with the positional preference.

Management of torticollis
Similar to congenital torticollis, conservative treatment until 6 months allows 90% of cases to self-resolve. Indications for surgical intervention include persistent torticollis >12 months or signs of facial hemi-hypoplasia. Despite surgical intervention, facial asymmetry will improve over years but may not completely resolve.

Cervical Lymphadenopathy

Lymphadenopathy of the neck manifests in the acute period as a reactive response usually to an upper respiratory tract or ear infection. This may be due to a bacterial, viral or mycobacterial cause. Palpable lymph nodes may be tender and are expected to resolve as the infection improves. Occasionally, reactive hyperplasia occurs as a non-tender mass with a non-specific cause.

Acute lymphadenopathy can progress to lymphadenitis when the lymph nodes become infected. Lymphadenitis requires rest and simple analgesia, and if precipitated by a bacterial infection, IV antibiotics are recommended. With IV antibiotics, lymphadenitis may progress into a lymph node abscess. These are typically seen in the 6-month to 3-year-old age group whereby the infected lymph node continues to enlarge despite antibiotics. They may be fluctuant on palpation, but deeper nodes may not be palpable. It is typically associated with superficial skin changes such as overlying erythema, and if left treated, an abscess may form. In cases of clinical uncertainty, an USS of the area may be used to assess an enlarged lymph node to look for evidence of a collection forming. Lymph node abscesses require an incision and drainage.

Mycobacterial Infections of the Head and Neck

Mycobacterial infections can be divided into tuberculosis and atypical (non-tuberculosis) mycobacteria. Atypical mycobacteria include *Mycobacterium avium-intracellulare*, *Mycobacterium scrofulaceum*, *Mycobacterium fortuitum* and *Mycobacterium chelonae*.

These infections are rarely seen in Western countries and are transmitted through oral ingestion of infected soil. Atypical mycobacterial lymphadenopathy is non-tender and affects lymph nodes of the cervical and submandibular chains higher up in the neck. Up to 50% of these infections with atypical mycobacterium subsequently form *cold abscesses*. As these lymph nodes tend to be deep, they do not display the expected superficial erythema or palpable fluctuance. Instead, atypical mycobacterial lymph node abscesses rupture in a collar-stud distribution within the subcutaneous space causing a superficial blue-purple discolouration. Overall, 10% of these then ulcerate to form multiple discharging sinuses at the skin.

Atypical mycobacterial lymph node abscesses respond poorly to antibiotics and require surgical excision of the lymph node. Their surgical management can be difficult, and different approaches have been advocated by some surgeons, particularly for MAIS lesions on the face where complete excision risks damage to the facial nerve.

In lymphadenopathy caused by tuberculosis, the condition is primarily a pulmonary infection which causes supraclavicular lymphadenopathy. Because of this, the typical management for non-TB mycobacterial lymphadenopathy differs from TB lymphadenopathy. TB responds well with chemotherapy over a span of 2 years whilst atypical mycobacterial lymphadenopathy requires surgical excision and could be considered for antibiotic treatment if an excision would be anatomically challenging – e.g. in a deep location or near the facial nerve.

Tuberculosis is the world's second leading infectious killer second to COVID-19. Multi-drug-resistant (MDR) TB is a public health crisis and poses a challenge for TB eradication. In Australia, there is a low incidence of TB; however, there is an over-representation of immigrants and First Nation's Australians. Epidemiological studies have found that the highest rates are found in children born overseas, and the annual notification rate was three times higher in First Nation's Australians compared to Australians not of First Nation background. Papua New Guinea (PNG) has been speculated to be epidemic with MDR TB and HIV. The cross-border spread into Australia from PNG is highlighted where 77% of paediatric TB cases in 2003–2012 were from PNG. Treatment outcomes for children of PNG heritage with TB in the Torres Strait were less favourable compared to Australian children. In a study evaluating transmission pathways within a community outbreak, cultural and family relationships were identified as key factors contributing to TB transmission. With a strong emphasis in cultural and family relationships in both First Nation Australian and PNG cultures, the elimination of TB becomes more difficult. Queensland faces a unique challenge in TB control compared to the rest of Australia given its proximity to PNG and First Nation Australian population, particularly in North Queensland. It is not unexpected that there is an over-representation of both cross-border and First Nation Australian children with TB.

Rarer Causes of Cervical Lymphadenopathy

Other conditions for consideration include cat scratch disease (*Bartonella henselae*), toxoplasmosis, Kawasaki disease and AIDS. Lymphadenopathy which persists in the subacute period (2–6 weeks) is likely to be viral. Viral lymphadenopathy like viral illnesses is treated with supportive measurements, such as rest, hydration and analgesia. Biopsies are indicated in cases of chronic lymphadenopathy (>6 weeks), an unclear diagnosis or when lymph nodes are >3 cm. Lymphadenopathy in the supraclavicular and posterior triangle are more concerning for malignancy or tuberculosis, whilst those located in the submandibular and anterior cervical are commonly infective.

MALIGNANCIES OF THE HEAD
AND NECK IN CHILDREN

Lymphoma

Lymphoma occurs when there is uncontrolled proliferation of lymphoid cells in lymphoid tissue. Primary causes of lymphoma are categorised as *Hodgkin's* and *non-Hodgkin's lymphoma* (*NHL*) which combined the third most common cause of cancer in adolescents.

NHL typically causes lymphadenopathy in the mediastinum (thymus) or abdomen. At the time of diagnosis, the child is usually symptomatic from nodal enlargement, and the NHL has likely spread to regional nodes and to other locations such as the neck or axilla. NHL responds well to chemotherapy and steroids. The surgical role of NHL is to aid in biopsy and cytological diagnosis rather than curative treatment.

HL originates in one group of lymph nodes and progresses following lymphatic pathways. Similar to NHL, surgery has limited involvement often only providing the tissue diagnosis in biopsies. Histologically, Reed–Sternberg cells are seen in HL. Surgical excision may be considered in certain cases whereby lymphoma is solely located in one area.

Cervical Rhabdomyosarcoma

Rhabdomyosarcoma is the most common form of sarcoma found in the paediatric population. It is usually diagnosed by the age of 14 and may be associated with familial syndromes – neurofibromatosis 1 and Li-Fraumeni. They arise from immature or satellite cells expected to become striated skeletal muscle cells but may also be found in atypical locations.

Within the neck, they may present as a painless mass with overlying skin changes. Occasionally, rhabdomyosarcomas may be suspected when a child presents with symptoms due to a mass effect on important structures. Excision of such lesions can be challenging due to its proximity to these structures and the overall cosmetic effect. Complete excision is typically recommended, but this should be conferred with a paediatric oncological specialist to discuss the role of chemotherapy or radiotherapy. Local lymph node biopsies may also be suggested in conjunction with imaging to determine the staging of a suspected rhabdomyosarcoma.

Secondary Malignancies

Secondary malignancies which may cause cervical lymphadenopathy include nasopharyngeal, thyroid neoplasms and neuroblastoma. These are present with hard and hyperplastic nodes which may be difficult to differentiate from reactive hyperplasia. Lymphadenopathies in these scenarios are biopsied for histopathological evaluation.

Skin Lesions of the Head and Neck

Pilomatrixoma or pilomatricoma, also known as calcifying epithelioma of Malherbe, is a benign tumour of hair follicles histologically defined by calcifications and ghost cells. It is the most common acquired soft tissue mass in children with 60–70% located in the head and neck. Pilomatrixomas are firm and non-tender mass that slowly grow and may be well circumscribed or irregular. They are located in the intradermal or subcutaneous space producing a white, yellow or blue discolouration superficially with no overlying punctum. These are typically seen as solitary lesions; however, in 2–3% of cases, multiple lesions are associated with Gardner's syndrome. Pilomatrixomas are managed with an excision which can occur under local anaesthetic for superficial lesions. As they do not have a capsule, rupture of the lesion during excision is not unexpected and does not predispose recurrence.

Summary

- Neck lumps are common in childhood.
- Anatomical location and history often point to the examination.
- Targeted radiological investigations are often helpful in confirming a diagnosis.
- It is important to formulate a differential diagnosis to guide investigations.

FURTHER READING

Bowling K, Hart N, Cox P, Srinivas G. Management of paediatric hernia. BMJ. 2017 October;359:j4484.

Hutson JM, Li R, Southwell BR, Newgreen D, Cousinery M. Regulation of testicular descent. Pediatr Surg Int. 2015 April;31(4):317–25.

Kim JS. Acute abdominal pain in children. Pediatr Gastroenterol Hepatol Nutr. 2013 December;16(4):219–24.

Reynolds S, Yap D, Marikar D, Roland D. Fifteen-minute consultation: The infant with a neck lump. Arch Dis Child Educ Pract Ed. 2020 October;105(5):258–61.

Velasquez J, Boniface MP, Mohseni M. Acute scrotum pain. [Updated 15 May 2022]. In: StatPearls [Internet]. Treasure Island (FL): StatPearls Publishing; 2022.

Managing Trauma in Tropical Queensland

8

Daniel Carroll

INTRODUCTION

Traumatic injuries remain the leading cause of avoidable death and injury during childhood. Between 2001 and 2012 (a 10-year period), there were 686,409 trauma-related hospitalisations in children in Australia. The total cost of child injury hospitalisations is estimated to be $212 million per year. Between 2016 and 2017, around 1.5% of children were hospitalised due to traumatic injury. Overall, boys were 1.5 times more likely than girls to be injured. Despite many attempts to reduce the incidence of these injuries, the number of patients presenting with traumatic injuries remains high and appears to be rising. However, there is some evidence that improvements have been made with a fall in the deaths from 6.2 deaths per 10,000 children in 2004–2006 to 4.1 deaths per 100,000 children in 2015–2017. The three leading causes of injury deaths in children were:

- Land transport accidents (29%)
- Accidental drowning (18%)
- Assault (11%)

It is clear that progress is being made in some major areas. In particular, in relation to road transport accidents, the reported death rate has more than halved between 2009 and 2018. The decline in road accident deaths has been mostly marked in children aged 0–4. The death rate due to accidental drowning has also shown some improvement between 2008–2010 and 2015–2017 with a 27% improvement during this time period. The rates of suicide and assault remain thankfully low although there has been little change over the same time period.

Despite these improvements in mortality, it would seem that the number of patients admitted to hospital with traumatic injuries over the same time period has gradually increased. It is important to reflect that the reported rate of hospitalised injuries is not uniform across Australia and it is almost twice as high in very remote areas compared to those seen in major cities.

The rate of hospitalised cases for assault was considerably higher in remote and very remote areas (87 and 50 per 100,000 children) compared with those seen in major cities (10 per 100,000). It is also higher in the lowest socioeconomic areas and considerably higher for indigenous children than the incidence reported in non-indigenous children. This remains a significant challenge among the population we service in North Queensland. Rates of hospitalisation for traumatic injuries are significant than those seen in metropolitan areas. Rural and remote residents in North Queensland are two to three times more likely

DOI: 10.1201/9781003156659-8

to suffer severe injuries than patients living in major cities. They are also five times more likely to die from their injuries. Urban-centric guidelines for treating trauma patients in transit to hospitals must be viewed with some caution as they are generally based on the 'scoop and run' principle. When aeromedical retrieval can take much longer such as in remote and very remote areas, it is more usual to consider starting treatment in a pre-hospital environment.

IMMEDIATE MANAGEMENT OF TRAUMATIC INJURIES

Despite the differences and difficulties encountered in our practice, the principles of trauma management remain the same as those utilised across all major trauma centres. The immediate management is summarised by the acronym **DRSCABCD**.

- **Danger**, e.g. traffic, powerlines, toxins, body fluids
  - If there is immediate threat to a patient's life and rapid movement is needed all efforts should be made to limit spinal movement without delaying treatment. It may be necessary to drag the patient using the ankle or arm/shoulder if alone.
  - High-voltage powerlines are very dangerous to rescuers. It is important to maintain a distance of 1 m per 10,000 V.
    - High voltage can cause instant death due to flash/arcing.
    - Electricity can travel through wet ground for many metres.
    - Do not get closer until the disconnection of power is confirmed.
  - Household electricity should be turned off and protected against being switched on again prior to rescue.
- **Response**
  - **Check if the casualty is responsive or unresponsive**.
    - Introduce yourself.
    - Gently shake the shoulder if a patient is not responsive.
    - **COWS**.
      - **C**an you hear me, **O**pen your eyes, **W**hat is your name, **S**queeze my hand.
- **Send for help**
  - Once you have made sure the area is safe and have determined if the patient is conscious or unconscious, it is time to call for help. If alone call 000.
  - Ideally one or more assistants are needed.
- **Catastrophic haemorrhage**
  - It is important to control catastrophic haemorrhage before checking the airway.
  - Do not remove penetrating objects as this can worsen haemorrhage.
  - Use direct firm pressure with hands and pads or bandages.
  - If unable to control, use either a **haemostatic dressing** or in a limb an **arterial tourniquet 5 cm above the injury/amputation**.
  - If not stopping, try a second tourniquet above the first.
  - **Record application time and tell retrieval team**.
  - Do not cover tourniquet with bandage/clothing.
- **Airway (and cervical spine)**
  - Look for signs of upper airway obstruction, e.g. use of accessory muscles.
  - Listen for upper airway noises and breath sounds.
  - Open the airway with the chin lift/jaw thrust manoeuvre.

It may be necessary to use an airway adjunct such as a Guedel airway when available to help secure the airway. It is important to remove loose foreign bodies and fluids from the mouth.

- **Maintain C-spine stability**
  - Support the head in a neutral position
  - Consider soft collar or sand/fluid bags and tape to support the neck
  - Need an assistant when removing a helmet to restrict movement
  - May need to position patient on the side to maintain airway
- **Breathing**
  - Expose the chest and assess respiratory effort, deformity, wounds
  - Inspect for respiratory effort and use of accessory muscles
  - Auscultate for breath sounds
- **Signs of tension pneumothorax**
  - Decreased/absent breath sounds
  - Hyper-resonance on percussion
  - Tachycardia, hypotension, dyspnoea
  - Distended neck veins

For Patients with Suspected Tension Pneumothorax Immediate Needle Decompression with a 14 G Needle Should Be Performed

For those patients with a sucking or open chest wound, a three-sided dressing should be applied. In general, the patients should be given supplemental oxygen to maintain saturations above 94% and bag-valve-mask ventilation may be required.

- **Circulation (and haemorrhage control)**
  - Assess heart rate and capillary refill time
  - Control external haemorrhage
  - Secure IV access (when not possible consider intraosseous access)

Where there are signs of **shock**, it is important to maintain tissue perfusion. IV fluids are given with an initial bolus of 10–20 mL/kg of warmed crystalloid. The patient is then reassessed.

- *Disability*: Basic neurological evaluation
  - **AVPU** (alert, voice, pain, unresponsive)
  - **Blood glucose level**
  - **Pupils** (size, reactivity, equal)

It is often impractical to get beyond these basic steps outside of the hospital environment; however, adopting a structured approach to the management of trauma has resulted in an improvement in outcomes for trauma patients. These steps are also sometimes referred to as the primary survey. The next stage in management is to move on to a more detailed assessment of the situation, the patient and further initiation of management. This is termed the 'secondary survey' and it is possible to continue the alphabetical theme by using the acronym **EFGHIJ** to remember the next important steps.

Secondary survey: EFGHIJ

Once the immediate lifesaving interventions and management have been initiated, it is possible to continue to more detailed clinical assessment.

- **(E) Exposure, environment and early notification and transfer**
  - Remove all clothing
  - Keep warm/prevent hypothermia
  - A rapid assessment of vital signs of injury and the mechanism of injury is made
    - The criteria for **early notification of trauma for transfer** are given in Table 8.1

TABLE 8.1   Physiological criteria for initiating early notification of trauma for transfer

VITAL SIGNS	ADULT	0–4 WEEKS	INFANT	1–8 YEARS	9–15 YEARS
RR/min	<10 or >30	<40 or >60	<20 or >50	<20 or >35	<15 or >25
SpO$_2$ on air	<90%	<95%	<95%	<95%	<95%
Systolic BP	<90	n/a	<60	<70	<80
HR/min	>120	<100 or >130	<90 or >170	<75 or >130	<65 or >120
Glasgow Coma Score (GCS)	<14	Altered LOC	Altered LOC	Altered LOC	Altered LOC

- **All penetrating injuries**
- **Blunt injuries with significant injuries or involving two or more regions**
  - Head/neck/chest/abdomen/pelvis/axilla
- **Specific injuries**
  - Limb amputation
  - Burns >20% adult; >10% child
  - Respiratory tract burns
  - Crush injury
  - Major compound fracture/open dislocation
  - Fracture to two or more long bones
  - Fracture pelvis
  - Suspected spinal cord injury
  - Life-threatening injuries
- **Mechanism of injury**
  - Ejection from vehicle
  - Motorcycle impact >30 kph
  - MVA >60 kph
  - Vehicle roll over
  - Pedestrian impact
  - Fall >3 m
  - Struck on head by object falling >3 m
  - Explosion

Any of the earlier-mentioned clinical scenarios are associated with a significant risk of life-threatening injuries and should be promptly referred to the local/state trauma escalation service. In Queensland, this is co-ordinated with RSQ (Retrieval Services Queensland).

- **(F) Full vital signs, FAST, family**
  - Check the vital signs, perform neurological observations, fontanelle in infants
  - Consider a FAST scan if appropriately trained and available
  - Communicate with family and friends
- **(G) Give pain relief, get resuscitation adjuncts**
  - Laboratory tests (FBC, UE, Lactate, troponin, BGL, LFT, group and hold, coags)
  - Monitor vital signs at least every 15 min
  - NGT or OGT for suspected base of skull fracture
  - Oxygen if indicated
  - Pain assessment and analgesia. Avoid opiates in head injuries
- **(H) History**
  - Allergies
  - Medications
  - Past medical history
  - Last meal
  - Events related to injury (mechanism, LOC, social issues)
- **(I) Head-to-toe (I)nspection**
  - General appearance
  - Head and face
  - Neck
  - Chest
  - Abdomen and flanks
  - Pelvis
  - Perineum/genitalia
  - Limbs
  - Inspect back
- **(J) Jot it down**
  - Ensure clear/contemporaneous documentation

Once the secondary survey has been completed, it is usually possible to set management priorities for patients and organise appropriate disposal of the patient to the correct setting. It is often the case that the secondary survey is completed over a longer period of time whilst resuscitation measures and communication with receiving centres and patient transport services are ongoing.

ABDOMINAL TRAUMA IN CHILDREN

Abdominal trauma is the commonest reason for referral to paediatric surgical services following trauma. Significant abdominal trauma is present in 25% of paediatric patients presenting with major trauma and is almost always blunt abdominal trauma (90% of cases). The assessment of the child with abdominal trauma is confounded by communication difficulties in younger children and pain, distress and other injuries often lead to injuries being missed on initial clinical assessment. Missed intra-abdominal injuries are the leading cause of avoidable death in children with traumatic injuries.

Clinical Assessment of the Child with Abdominal Injuries

A careful physical examination should be conducted, where possible the child should be kept warm and comfortable and comforted by parents or other caregivers. Frightened and distressed children are very difficult to assess. It is important to complete the primary and secondary surveys as well as ensure that children are adequately resuscitated before trying to make a more detailed assessment of the abdomen. Assessment begins by taking a detailed history where possible determining the mechanism of injury and taking a careful handover from first responders. It is important to remember that children are at higher risk than adult patients from blunt abdominal trauma as the abdominal musculature is less well developed and solid organs such as the spleen and liver are relatively larger and prone to damage. Non-accidental injuries can cause massive damage to solid organs and bowel perforation with relatively few external signs of bruising.

Inspection of the abdomen and flanks to look for signs of seatbelt injuries and obvious bruising or grazing is the first step. Children restrained by seatbelts often have a mark in high-speed collisions. Bruising of the flanks and umbilicus can be seen several hours after an injury with retroperitoneal bleeding.

Gentle abdominal examination with warm hands and in a systematic manner can reveal areas of focal tenderness. Particular care must be given to examining bony prominences, including the ribs as well as palpating both kidneys. Deeper palpation may be necessary to demonstrate tenderness associated with an injury to a solid organ, but sometimes clinical examination is remarkably benign even with significant underlying injuries. Listening for bowel sounds is sometimes performed but has little clinical value. Pain on movement is often significant and the child may remain still to minimise peritoneal irritation if there is either a hollow viscus or solid organ injury. Careful attention must be given to the vital signs as early signs of deterioration are subtle in children and the only consistent feature prior to decompensation may be a tachycardia.

A number of investigations are useful in completing an assessment for abdominal injuries. Even in patients with few clinical signs, a history of significant trauma should lead to some baseline investigations which have been described earlier as parts of the secondary survey. In addition to these tests, it is useful to carefully check a urine specimen. In critically unwell children, then a catheter may have been inserted. The presence of macroscopic haematuria is often significant as there is a high rate of solid organ injury in children with macroscopic haematuria. Plain abdominal radiographs usually add little to the assessment, but bedside ultrasound scanning can often demonstrate free fluid. It is important to remember that many significant injuries are missed on ultrasound scan assessments in children. Patients with either a significant mechanism of injury or clinical signs should undergo more detailed examinations using cross-sectional imaging. Whilst we adopt an as low as reasonably achievable as low as reasonably achievable (ALARA) approach to ordering radiological investigations, a CT scan is often the only practical way to rule out significant intra-abdominal injuries. If the child has other injuries such as a head injury with reduced level of consciousness, it may be necessary to exclude life-threatening intra-abdominal injuries prior to embarking upon lengthy operative procedures as deterioration intra-operatively from an intra-abdominal cause can be catastrophic.

It is important to involve the radiologist to ensure that the imaging is performed in such a way as to get the most information from the least amount of radiation. Cross-sectional imaging with CT scan remains the gold standard investigation for the management of traumatic injuries in children but duodenal and other retroperitoneal injuries may not be visible on early imaging and so delayed imaging may be required if children continue to exhibit clinical signs of peritonism. Careful observation and frequent reassessment are required for patients admitted with significant abdominal trauma.

Assessment of the Child with Delayed Presentation

It is often the case that a child in North Queensland is assessed initially in a remote or very remote area. Once transfer has been completed it may be many hours or even days since the original injury. At this stage, it is unlikely that these patients have major solid organ injury and it may be possible to adopt a more conservative approach to imaging. If this strategy is adopted, it is important to admit and observe these patients as often subtle signs such as a minor tachycardia can be the only sign that significant underlying injury exists. In general, it is more usual to treat these patients as if they were presenting acutely and perform a dose-limited CT scan. These patients require discussion with senior clinicians to achieve the optimal strategy.

Management of Blunt Abdominal Trauma

Patients who are haemodynamically unstable despite attempts at resuscitation and those with obvious perforation may require urgent surgical intervention without radiological assessment. Fortuitously, this group of patients is very rare; it is almost always possible to proceed with radiological investigation and complete assessment before progressing to theatre for a damage control laparotomy. This is often done with the support of PICU and anaesthesia and ED colleagues with continued resuscitation continuing during transport both to and from the CT scanner. An understanding of the injuries present prior to embarking upon the laparotomy increases the surgeon's ability to quickly and efficiently deal with problems encountered as well as allowing for operative planning. A detailed description of the steps necessary in performing a damage control laparotomy is beyond the scope of this book, but essentially a midline incision is used and all four quadrants of the abdomen are packed to control bleeding and establish haemodynamic stability as quickly as possible. Once control of the situation has been achieved, a detailed inspection of each quadrant is made until all bleeding is controlled. It is sometimes necessary to pause at this stage to allow for blood products to be delivered and help to arrive. For patients with major injuries, it is possible to leave the abdominal compartment unclosed and return the patient to PICU for continued support prior to performing more definitive surgery. Radiological assessment at this stage can be helpful and some injuries can be managed by interventional radiology techniques.

The vast majority of patients with a mechanism of blunt abdominal trauma can be managed conservatively. Paediatric surgery has been at the forefront of adopting a conservative strategy for the management of abdominal trauma, and children require intervention far less than adult patients with similar injuries. In the 2000 American Paediatric Surgery Association (APSA) guidelines, non-operative management of liver and spleen injuries became the standard of care. Solid organ injuries were classified as Grades 1–5 and patients are generally admitted for observation for a period of time dictated by the grade of injury. The commonest strategy employed was grade of injury +2 days for bedrest and observation followed by a period of risk reduction in activities for 6 weeks to 3 months. In patients who have been transferred from remote or very remote areas, it may be necessary to adopt a more cautious strategy particularly in regard to avoiding subsequent trauma.

THORACIC TRAUMA IN CHILDREN

Major thoracic trauma is uncommon in paediatric trauma reported in between 5 and 12% of paediatric admissions with traumatic injuries. It is important, as it is associated with higher morbidity and mortality than that seen with other types of injuries. The relative rarity of these injuries increases the complexity of management; they should be managed in consultation with a paediatric surgeon.

Clinical Presentation

Children who have experienced major trauma can present in a variety of ways ranging from chest wall or intrapleural injuries (rib fractures, flail chest, pneumothorax) to lung, mediastinal (heart/trachea/oesophagus) or diaphragmatic injuries.

Differences in Anatomy and Physiology

The chest wall is more compliant in children and the thickness and protection offered by the muscular layers is reduced compared to adults. The thoracic organs are subsequently more likely to be damaged in children than adults. It is important to remember that the relative elasticity of the thorax means that rib fractures when they do occur are associated with a much higher risk of significant injury. Children are at greater risk of physiological embarrassment following chest trauma as they have a smaller physiological reserve with a relatively diminished functional residual capacity and higher metabolic rate with a higher oxygen requirement.

Management of Thoracic Trauma in Children

Initial management

The initial management of thoracic trauma shares the common pathway for all trauma outlined previously. APLS guidelines suggest a chest radiograph as first-line imaging in patients with major trauma and this can be useful in identifying patients with major injuries. Most patients with a history of major trauma will require cross-sectional imaging to identify the extent of any intrathoracic injuries and it may be possible to avoid the added radiation burden of the initial chest radiograph if further imaging is likely to be necessary. For patients with suspected life-threatening injuries such as tension pneumothorax, it is unwise to perform radiological investigations prior to patient stabilisation and initiation of management as deterioration in the radiology department is a potential problem and should be avoided.

Patterns of Injury

The most common injury recorded in children admitted to hospital with traumatic injuries of the chest is pulmonary contusion. This is recorded in over 50% of cases. This can be seen on a simple chest radiograph and can be identified clinically by an area of abnormal auscultation, respiratory distress, localised tenderness and rarely haemoptysis. Subsequent consolidation can result in pneumonia in 20% of patients with ARDS being seen in up to 20% of patients. Occasionally, alveolar disruption can lead to pneumothorax, pneumatocele and surgical emphysema.

The second most common injury is pneumothorax which is observed as an isolated injury in up to 30% of cases of major blunt thoracic trauma. Minor pneumothoraces (<20% of the hemithorax) usually resolve spontaneously and do not require drainage. A large pneumothorax can result in respiratory distress and ventilatory failure. Clinically the affected hemithorax is hyper-resonant to percussion with reduced breath sounds. **In the presence of a tension pneumothorax, the mediastinum is displaced to the contralateral side with impairment of venous return**. This is a surgical emergency and should be drained immediately and prior to further imaging studies. Tension pneumothorax is more common in children than adults because of the higher mobility of mediastinal structures.

Haemothorax is the third most common complication of blunt thoracic trauma in children. It is most commonly caused by laceration of the lung parenchyma with a rib fracture. It is associated with a high-mortality rate and can lead to significant blood loss. It should be managed immediately to reduce the risk of hypovolemic shock, lung volume loss, empyema and lung entrapment.

Mediastinal injuries include damage to the great vessels, tracheal and bronchial injuries, heart injuries and oesophageal and diaphragmatic rupture. These injuries are rare but are potentially lethal (around 1/3 in the first hour following injury).

Imaging in Thoracic Trauma in Children

Radiological evaluation is fundamental to the successful management of thoracic trauma in children. It is well established that children are relatively more sensitive to the risks of ionising radiation than their adult counterparts due to their higher cell division rate and longer life expectancy. This is particularly true in younger children but in general children are roughly four times more sensitive to ionising radiation. The ALARA principle has been applied to most pathways for guiding radiological investigations in children.

No consensus has been reached for the optimal imaging strategy for thoracic trauma and in general decisions should be guided by senior clinicians when there are uncertainties surrounding the correct timing and modality of imaging to be used.

Patient scenarios are often significantly more complex than simple algorithms can effectively account for, and this is particularly true for our patients in North Queensland. Extended transfer times and the need for multiple reassessments mean that our patients are significantly different in terms of presentation to those larger series reported in the literature. In general, children with major polytrauma (particularly those with major head injuries or requiring theatre management) will require cross-sectional imaging. This should be guided by careful consultation with the radiology department to ensure that adequate images are captured to answer the appropriate clinical questions that may be posed. Ultrasound scan assessment of thoracic injuries is somewhat limited, and the use of MRI imaging is often impractical in critically unwell children. In practice, critically unwell children require CT scanning and often this is performed as part of a 'pan-scan' where a CT is taken to exclude injuries in multiple areas at the same time. Limiting the transfers from a high-dependency area to the radiology department is useful in reducing risk to the patients should they deteriorate.

In practice, first-line imaging is usually a chest radiograph taken in the emergency bay. The dose of radiation is very low (roughly 0.02 mSv). Image interpretation is often more difficult because the film is taken as a supine anteroposterior image. Despite this, the chest radiograph can be useful in order to make further decisions whilst considering the next management steps. In large studies in metropolitan patients looking at paediatric patients presenting with thoracic trauma, a normal chest radiograph is associated with an exceptionally low rate of subsequent clinically important findings on CT scan. This is not always true in our cohort of patients who have significantly higher acuity of injuries. Generally, a careful assessment of the patient, including a detailed history, is required to guide the optimal strategy for imaging. Often these decisions are best made in direct consultation with the team who will be managing the patient once admitted.

CT scan should be performed in all cases with suspected pneumomediastinum or thoracic spine injuries.

Management of Paediatric Thoracic Trauma

It is often appropriate to manage paediatric thoracic trauma following adult guidelines. The majority of patients are managed conservatively. Pulmonary contusions are treated with adequate analgesia and careful monitoring to ensure adequate oxygenation and gas exchange. The use of epidural catheters and intercostal nerve block are often helpful. In patients with severe trauma, mechanical ventilation may be necessary, and if a patient is ventilated, this is often a good time to institute a nerve block.

Pneumothorax and haemothorax are often managed conservatively. This is particularly true for patients in whom the initial chest radiograph is normal. In the case of a large pneumothorax (>20% of the hemithorax) or haemothorax, an intercostal catheter is required to drain the collection of air or blood. An estimation of the appropriate size of the intercostal catheter is four times the correct size of endotracheal tube for the patient, although larger bore tubes may be required for adequate drainage of a haemothorax. Ideally the intercostal catheter should not be too large as this causes increased pain and subsequent reduced chest movements limit ventilation. For patients with prolonged pneumothorax and air leak, we should consider the possibility of a bronchopleural fistula or a major airway injury and further imaging may be required. Fortunately, the majority of these cases settle spontaneously with conservative strategies.

Patients with pneumomediastinum should have targeted imaging to rule out oesophageal or tracheo-bronchial injuries. They may require prolonged conservative management with nasogastric feeding and empirical antimicrobial therapy. Follow-up imaging is almost always required.

HEAD INJURIES IN CHILDREN

Head injuries are a common cause at hospital accounting for up to 2% of all presentations to specialist children's emergency services in Australia. Although most are minor, head injuries remain a significant cause of morbidity and mortality. It is important to have a framework for identifying and appropriately managing children with head injuries both as isolated injuries and also in the context of polytrauma. The vast majority of patients with minor head injury do not require anything other than careful assessment and observation. Several 'clinical decision rules' are used to determine patients who require further investigation, e.g. CT scanning.

CDR in the Management of Paediatric Head Injury

A number of high-quality clinical decision rule systems are available to guide decision-making. The three most commonly used are PECARN (US), CHALICE (UK) and CATCH (Canada). CHALICE is most useful for the higher-risk cohort with GCS <13. Some common themes exist between all these Clinical Decision Rules (CDRs) and a fuller exploration of them is beyond the scope of this chapter.

In general, children with a GCS <14, or with altered mental status or a palpable skull fracture, should have a CT scan. If there is a witnessed loss of consciousness greater than 5 s or a severe mechanism of injury or abnormal behaviour, they should also be given prompt consideration of a CT scan.

CHALICE CDR Summary

A CT scan is required if any of the following are present:

History:

- Witnessed LOC >5 min
- Amnesia >5 min
- Abnormal drowsiness
- >Three vomits
- Suspicion of Non-accidental injury (NAI)
- Seizures

Examination:

- GCS <14 or <15 in patients <1 year of age
- Suspicion of penetrating or depressed skull fracture
- Tense fontanelle
- Signs of basal skull fracture
- Positive focal neurology
- Presence of a haematoma or laceration >5 cm if <1 year old

Mechanism:

- High-speed road traffic accident (RTA) (>64 km/h)
- Fall >3 m height
- High-speed injury from projectile or object

Patients requiring CT scanning should be referred for assessment to the neurosurgical team to allow for appropriate planning and transfer arrangements to be made if necessary.

Concurrent investigation management and referral may be required for the child with significant head injuries. These are often seen in the context of polytrauma and a co-ordinated team response is required to ensure the best outcomes for these patients. Management aims to maintain adequate cerebral perfusion and oxygenation.

Management of Children with High-Risk Head Injuries and Other Life-Threatening Injuries

Children with significant polytrauma and associated severe head injuries require urgent paediatric critical care/neurosurgical advice. Paediatric surgeons often find themselves in a position of assessing and co-ordinating care in patients with polytrauma in conjunction with ED and retrieval colleagues. Priorities in management are:

- ABC assessment and management
- Active management of raised intra-cranial pressure (ICP)
- Consideration of other serious injuries
- Frequent clinical reassessment
- Urgent CT scan or urgent transfer as required

Management of Raised ICP

Effective management of raised ICP helps maintain adequate cerebral perfusion, which can be summarised as follows.

Airway and Breathing

- Maintain the airway with cervical spine precautions.
- Avoid hypercarbia and hypoxia.
- Rapid sequence induction is recommended for intubation.

Circulatory Support

- Maintain adequate blood pressure and tissue perfusion.

Positioning

- Raise head of bed 20–30 degrees.

Hyperosmolar Agents

- Mannitol and 3% NaCl may be used under guidance from PICU/neurosurgery.

General Measures

- Actively manage seizures
- Provide adequate analgesia and sedation
- Avoid hyperthermia
- Consider neuromuscular blockade
- Antiemetics should be considered prior to transfer

MANAGEMENT OF ORTHOPAEDIC INJURIES

Orthopaedic injuries are common in the child with polytrauma. Around 75% of children with poly-trauma have orthopaedic injuries. Central musculoskeletal injuries increase intensive care and length of hospital stay and their early recognition and management improve outcomes. Skeletal trauma is rarely life-threatening but can be a significant cause of long-term morbidity.

Initial Assessment

Immediate assessment follows the principles of trauma management outlined previously. Younger chil-dren have a relatively large head compared to adults and are at greater risk of cervical spine injury. Because they have relative lax ligaments, they are prone to cervical spine injury without radiological abnormality (SCIWORA) and MRI may be required to recognise these injuries. It is important to protect the cervical spine during assessment.

Open Fractures

Open fractures are classified according to the Gustilo–Anderson classification. Wound debridement should be ideally carried out by an orthopaedic surgeon in all open fractures. This should be carried out within 24 h whenever possible, unless there is gross contamination of wounds, devascularisation of the limb or compartment syndrome in which case it should be carried out more urgently.

Compartment syndrome

A high index of clinical suspicion needs to be maintained to avoid preventable injury in the context of compartment syndrome. Children tend to develop swelling and compartment syndrome later than adults. The 5 Ps (pain, pallor, paraesthesia, paralysis and pulselessness) are less reliable in children than the 3 As:

- Analgesia requirement
- Anxiety
- Agitation

Repeated clinical examination is the key to early diagnosis. If compartment syndrome is suspected, intra-compartment pressure should be measured. If compartment syndrome is suspected, then urgent orthopaedic evaluation and consideration of fasciotomies are mandated.

CHALLENGES FOR THE FUTURE

Trauma remains one of the leading causes for death and subsequent disability in children. This is particularly true in developing countries and there is a higher burden of traumatic injury in children in remote and rural communities. A full exploration of the incidence of trauma in tropics has not been carried out, although early evidence from databases suggest that the rate of major trauma in both children and adults is higher in non-metropolitan areas. It will be essential to construct databases to keep records of patients injured in trauma with reference to location to allow for prevention and management strategies to be improved.

FURTHER READING

Babl FE, Borland ML, Phillips N, Kochar A, Dalton S, McCaskill M, et al. Accuracy of PECARN, CATCH, and CHALICE head injury decision rules in children: A prospective cohort study. Lancet. 2017;389(10087): 2393–402.

Cullen PM. Paediatric trauma. Contin Educ Anaesth Crit Care Pain Med. 2012;12(3):157–61.

Lynch T, Kilgar J, Al Shibli A. Pediatric abdominal trauma. Curr Pediatr Rev. 2018;14(1):59–63.

Reynolds SL. Pediatric thoracic trauma: Recognition and management. Emerg Med Clin North Am. 2018 May;36(2): 473–83.

Paediatric Burns

9

Helen Buschel and Daniel Carroll

Burns in children are common with nearly 10,000 cases managed by burn units across Australia and New Zealand each year. In our unit in Northern Australia, we receive around 250–300 new referrals every year for paediatric patients with burns. Understanding the pathophysiology and management of burns is critical to reducing potential long-term physical and psychological consequences as well as reducing the need for surgery. The management of burns in a child involves a multi-disciplinary team, including paediatric surgeons, occupational therapists, physiotherapists, dieticians, nursing staff, social workers, indigenous liaison officers and psychologists. The key to better outcomes in burn management is the correct early treatment of a burn to minimise tissue damage and reduce the need for surgical intervention.

EPIDEMIOLOGY

About two-thirds of paediatric burns occur in children less than 5 years of age. The pattern of injury in children differs from that seen in adults with the most common mechanism being scald (over 50%) followed by contact, flame and friction. Other mechanisms, including chemical, radiant heat, electrical and pressurised gas/air, are uncommon causes of burns in children. A recent study of burns in children in Australia identified over 25,000 patients admitted to hospital between 2002 and 2012. Children from the ages of 1 to 5 years have the highest incidence of admission to hospital with burns (around 1:1000). The estimated cost of burn injuries in children over this 10-year period was around $168 million.

It has been reported that in tropical, rural and remote areas, the pattern is again different with increasing incidence of contact and flame burns compared to the metropolitan centres of Australia and New Zealand. This is in keeping with the demographic of this population where activities involving campfires and unshielded exhaust (mufflers) in motorbikes and quadbikes are more common and are of significance as these burns are more likely to be deep when compared to scald burns.

PATHOPHYSIOLOGY

As healthy organic tissue is exposed to thermal injury, tissue damage occurs. At temperatures above 43°C, protein denaturation begins to occur; at temperatures above 45°C, permanent cell damage occurs. The damage to tissues results in complex effects on the damaged cells, resulting in cytokine release causing profound intracellular and extracellular changes in tissue perfusion and initiation of fluid movement from the intracellular and intravascular compartments to the extravascular space. Burns may be associated with

DOI: 10.1201/9781003156659-9

local and systemic effects. The three zones of tissue damage and the potential for recovery in each of these zones were first articulated by Jackson in 1947. He proposed three zones of injury:

- the zone of coagulation
- zone of stasis and
- zone of hyperaemia

The zone of coagulation is the central aspect of the burn where there is maximal damage and irreversible tissue necrosis. The zone of stasis surrounds this area and is potentially reversible with adequate first aid and resuscitation. Optimal management of the burn over subsequent days may prevent the zone of stasis from progressing to necrosis and tissue loss. The outer zone of hyperaemia is characterised by a reactive hyper-perfusion of the tissue. Although this model has proved useful in terms of dictating our response to burn injuries, this is probably an overly simplistic and reductionist model of what is happening at a cellular level, and it is now thought that significantly more tissue than previously considered salvageable is able to be preserved.

The systemic response to a burn is typically significant in burns greater than 10% of total body surface area (TBSA) in children and is the result of inflammatory mediators, including cytokines, thromboxane A1 and bradykinin. Organ systems that may be affected include:

- *Cardiovascular*: Hypovolaemia secondary to increased capillary permeability with loss of protein and fluid into the interstitial space and myocardial damage from toxins. In large burns, myocardial contractility may become depressed. Red cells may be directly destroyed by the burn.
- *Pulmonary*: Respiratory failure secondary to pulmonary oedema and/or acute respiratory distress syndrome, even where there is no inhalation injury. In cases of smoke inhalation, bronchoconstriction and respiratory distress syndrome may occur.
- *Gastrointestinal*: Dysmotility, ileus and malabsorption. Peripheral and splanchnic vasoconstrictions occur in larger burns. Atrophy of small bowel mucosa occurs.
- *Renal*: Secondary to hypovolaemia, decreased renal perfusion and renal damage secondary to myoglobin.
- *Immune system*: Decreased white cell function, decreased globulins thereby decreased immunity.

PATIENT ASSESSMENT AND EARLY MANAGEMENT

Primary Survey

In children, nearly 90% of burns are less than 10% TBSA, and the majority do not require immediate lifesaving intervention and resuscitation. All burns should receive appropriate first aid which involves:

- Removing any source of ongoing burn (extinguish flames, remove hot clothing and/or irrigate chemicals) and
- **Cooling the burn surface with 20 minutes of cool running water (effective within 3-hour post-burn)**

Appropriate first aid reduces burn progression and allows for recovery of tissue that is in the zone of stasis and zone of hyperaemia and is analgesic. Children should be monitored for evidence of hypothermia. Ice should not be used as this can result in further tissue damage by reducing the blood supply to damaged tissues.

Large burns require emergent primary and secondary surveys with simultaneous assessment and resuscitation. The airway should be assessed and can be threatened acutely secondary to inhalation injury (inhalation of hot gases or products of combustion) and over the following hours secondary to oedema. Features concerning for an impending loss of airway include:

- History of burn in an enclosed space
- Associated explosion
- Facial burns
- Singed facial hairs
- Dysphonia
- Hoarse cough
- Stridor
- Respiratory distress

Any acute airway concerns should be managed with high-flow oxygen, securing a definitive airway and appropriate respiratory support. Assessment of adequacy of breathing involves the measurement of oxygen saturation, respiratory rate, chest wall expansion and identification of circumferential chest wall burns impacting respiration that may require escharotomy (see next). Large burns are associated with significant fluid sequestration and loss which can result in hypovolaemia. Haemodynamic status should be promptly assessed; two large bore cannulas should be placed (in non-burnt skin where possible) and fluid resuscitation should be commenced.

The fluid needs of the child with a burn greater than 10% TBSA can be calculated using the Parklands formula:

- **2–4 mL crystalloid × kg body weight × TBSA plus maintenance fluids (with dextrose).**

Half of this volume is given in the first 8 hours and the remainder in the following 16 hours, starting from the time of injury. This formula should act as a guideline, and further fluid resuscitation may be required based on urine output (aim greater than 1 mL/kg/hour), and therefore, an indwelling urinary catheter should be inserted to allow for hourly urine output to be monitored.

Assessing TBSA

There are multiple methods of assessing burn TBSA in children. For smaller burns, the palmar surface is used and represents about 1% TBSA. For larger burns, the paediatric rule of nines can be used. For older children, this rule is the same as in adults: head (9%), upper limbs (9% each), lower limbs (18% each), anterior trunk (18%), posterior trunk (18%), neck (1%) and genitalia/perineum (1%). To modify for children less than 10 years of age, 0.5% is taken from each leg and added to the head (1%) for each year of life after 12 months. For more accurate calculations, Lund–Browder burn diagrams should be used. A modified Lund–Browder chart can be seen in Figure 9.1. In real-life situations, it is often challenging to accurately determine the TBSA of burn; this is particularly true for patients with darker skin as we have

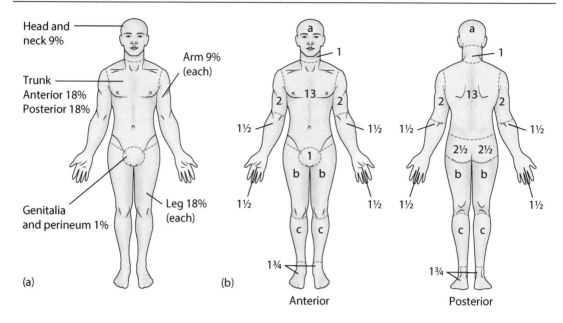

FIGURE 9.1   Modified Lund–Browder chart for burn TBSA estimation in children.

	0 yr	1 yr	5 yr	10 yr	15 yr
Relative percentage of body surface areas (% BSA) affected by growth					
a— ½ of head	9½	8½	6½	5½	4½
b— ½ of 1 thigh	2¾	3¼	4	4¼	4½
c— ½ of 1 lower leg	2½	2½	2¾	3	3¼

identified a large number of patients with significant underestimates of TBSA burn with darkly coloured skin; if the blistered epithelium is not removed, then the skin changes can be subtle and easily missed on photographs or on direct inspection of the skin.

Although estimation of TBSA is useful in determining the need for transfer and higher-level support for patients, it is frequently over- or under-estimated. I usually recommend that referring clinicians with smartphone access download the NSW ITIM application. This has a section for paediatric burn estimation as well as calculating fluid requirements. After inputting the patient's weight and age and drawing the distribution of burns on an avatar it is possible to accurately estimate TBSA even from photographs or for teams with little specialist knowledge in burn surgery who are unfamiliar with Lund–Browder chart.

Assessing Burn Depth

Although burn depth assessment can be inaccurate in the early stages, it is an important aspect of early management. Burns are typically divided into three categories based upon the depth of the injury (see Figure 9.2).

- Superficial
- Partial thickness (superficial dermal and mid-dermal)
- Deep burns (deep dermal and full thickness)

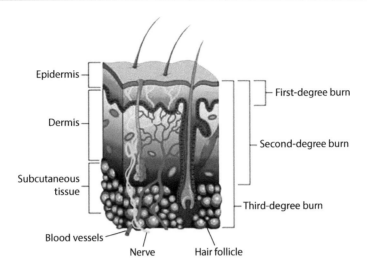

FIGURE 9.2 Schematic showing different parts of skin involved in different depth burns.

Superficial burns (previously called 'first-degree burns') involve the epidermis only and present as painful erythema without blistering. Superficial burns are not included in the TBSA calculation. They are typically associated with sunburn and minor scald burns. These burns tend to be painful and heal quickly with moisturiser alone without causing scarring.

Partial-thickness burns ('second-degree burns') are divided into superficial dermal and mid-dermal. They range from pale pink to dark pink in colour, have associated blistering and are typically painful with present blanching. Partial-thickness burns typically heal without scarring with appropriate first aid and regular dressings. However, some mid-dermal burns may progress, particularly if there is ongoing tissue injury (e.g. inappropriate or inadequate first aid or subsequent infection).

Deep burns ('third-degree burns') are the most severe burns and typically cause significant scarring if left to heal spontaneously over a prolonged period of time. Various studies have demonstrated that wounds that take over 14 days to heal completely are associated with a much higher risk of problematic scarring, and it is important that treatment is guided to try and ensure that burns heal as quickly as possible to minimise the risk of the need for scar management. Deep burns can be further divided into deep dermal and full-thickness burns. Features to distinguish deep burns from more superficial burns include:

- **Absent sensation**
- **Blanching**

Deep dermal burns may have some blistering and appear 'blotchy red' in colour secondary to extravasation of haemoglobin from red cell damage. Full-thickness burns are typically pale white. Common causes of deep burns include:

- Contact burns (particularly with motorbike mufflers),
- Flame burns
- Electrical burns
- Some scald injuries particularly in infants

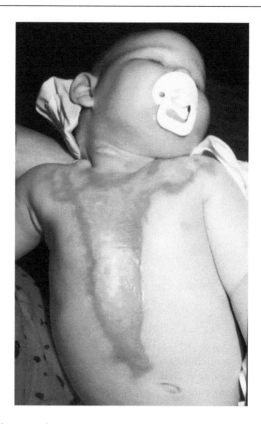

FIGURE 9.3   Full-thickness burn to chest.

Some deep burns extend beyond the dermis to the subcutaneous tissues; this is typically seen in friction burns. Deep burns typically require surgical management and long-term scar management. The dead and devitalised tissue should be removed as soon as practical to allow healing to commence and reduce the risk of subsequent infection which delays the healing process.

Unfortunately for clinicians, most burns exhibit a combination of different depths of burns in an unpredictable fashion. An example of a child with a combination of partial-thickness and full-thickness burns from a scald can be seen in Figure 9.3.

Completing the Primary Survey

Other important steps in early management of large burns include:

- Keeping the patient warm (including warm fluids and room temperature)
- Analgesia
- Nasogastric tube insertion (this is particularly important in patients requiring aeromedical retrieval)

Following the primary survey, a secondary survey should be performed paying attention to involvement of special areas including the eyes, perineum and genitals. The limbs should be assessed for circumferential burns and impending neurovascular compromise that may require urgent escharotomy. A history including vaccination status (for tetanus) should also be obtained.

Management of Burns

Escharotomy

For children with circumferential, deep burns, the thick overlying eschar can result in reduced venous drainage and ultimately impair arterial flow to the limbs/digits. Full-thickness chest burns can also impair ventilation. Associated oedema secondary to tissue injury and resuscitation can worsen swelling and venous drainage; ultimately, accumulation of fluid underneath the inelastic eschar affects arterial flow, resulting in absent distal pulses by palpation and/or Doppler examination. In such cases, emergency escharotomy should be performed. This involves an incision made on the medial and lateral aspects of the extremity. The depth of the incision should extend to the subcutaneous tissue. When the hands are involved, escharotomy incisions should be extended over the thenar and hypothenar eminences and/or the dorsolateral aspects of the digits. Although confronting, there is usually minimal bleeding as this is a full-thickness injury. It is important to look for signs of ischaemic-reperfusion injury. If increased compartment pressures are noted, fasciotomies should be performed. The scarring after escharotomies can be extensive and is often hypertrophic. A representation of the correct site for incisions can be seen in Figure 9.4.

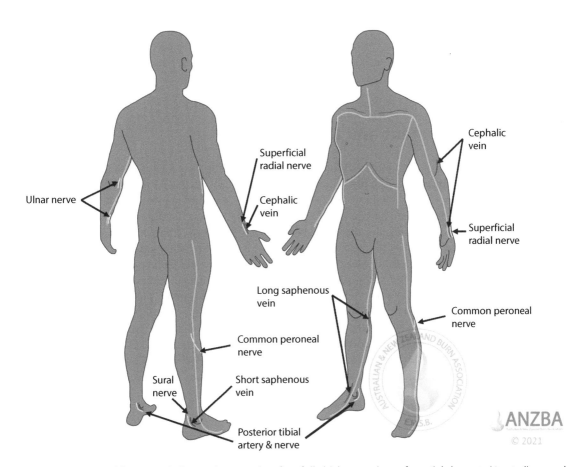

FIGURE 9.4 Incisions used for escharotomies for full-thickness circumferential burns. (Australian and New Zealand Burn Association Ltd [ANZBA] (2022). Emergency Management of Severe Burns course manual (version 19). © Copyright, Australian and New Zealand Burn Association. Produced with permission.) *(Continued)*

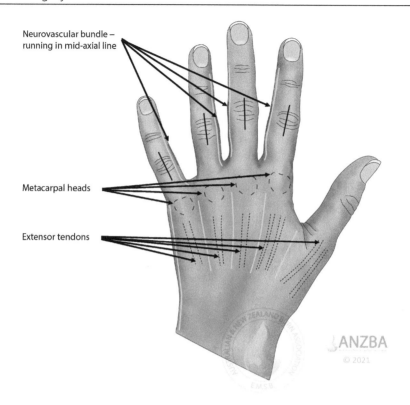

Neurovascular bundle – running in mid-axial line

Metacarpal heads

Extensor tendons

FIGURE 9.4   *(Continued)*

Wound Management and Dressings

There are a large number of commonly used dressings for burns in children. Superficial burns can typically be managed with regular moisturiser, medicinal honey or Solugel alone. Partial-thickness and deep burns require regular dressings and wound review. The preferred dressings are impregnated with silver (which has a strong antimicrobial action) and include Mepilex Ag and Acticoat. Both dressings can be placed on a clean burn, secured with an adhesive sheet (e.g. Hypafix) and left for 3–5 days. Silver dressings have the added benefit of antimicrobial activity and have been shown to improve healing time in partial-thickness burns. In Tropical North Queensland, we generally advocate for the use of Mepilex Ag as the first choice of dressings for burns. It has the significant advantage over Acticoat in that it does not need to be kept moist which can be challenging for families, Acticoat loses its antimicrobial action if not kept moist.

Silver sulfadiazine (SSD) cream is commonly used in adults but not typically recommended for children. SSD cream requires daily changing which involves removing all of the cream from the burn and re-applying; this can be a painful process for children and increases anxiety related to dressing changes. Most partial-thickness burns will heal within 14 days with minimal to no scarring. Continuous reassessment of burn depth is required to determine which burns are healing and which are likely to require surgical intervention.

> **Effective wound management with adequate initial cleaning and debridement of the burn with subsequent appropriate wound management with dressings is the cornerstone in preventing avoidable morbidity in burns. It significantly reduces the need for burn grafting which is both costly and has high short- and long-term morbidities for children and their families.**

In an attempt to try and optimise burn management in North Queensland, we offer a 24-hour burn service where we frequently give advice on the management of all burns within the region to try and ensure that management is optimal. We receive referrals via an email-based system directing referring clinicians to contact the team, and then we provide immediate real-time advice on managing the injury including follow-up arrangements.

Operative Management

Deep burns often require both emergent and non-emergent operative management, which may include:

- Debridement
- Excision
- Skin grafting and/or
- Placement of a matrix
- Escharotomies
- Fasciotomies

Occasionally, there are small, thin, full-thickness burns that are not suitable for grafting, which can be excised and primarily closed. For larger areas, the most common management is debridement and a split-thickness skin graft. The burn eschar is typically debrided in theatre, which may be done using various instruments, including a scalpel, the dermatome, a Weck knife or hydrosurgery system (for example Versajet).

A split-thickness skin graft is then harvested, most commonly from the thigh or buttock and secured to the healthy wound bed using sutures, surgical staples or skin glue, e.g. Histoacryl. For the most severe burns where there is significant tissue loss, a temporising matrix may be used in the first instance, and a graft placed at a later date.

Often in children following grafting, a thermoplastic splint is used to reduce movement of the affected area and allow healing of the graft. The key principles in burn surgery are to:

- Prevent further tissue loss (remove devitalised tissue to prevent infection)
- Create a healthy environment for healing (ensure adequate blood supply)
- Prevent subsequent infection (application of antimicrobial dressings)
- Allow grafted skin cells to establish themselves (prevent shear forces/immobilise wound)

Principles of Wound Dressings

Repeated experimental models have demonstrated the importance of the microenvironment in wound healing. Wounds are thought to heal best in a moist environment. In the early stages of wound healing, the tissues are fragile. For optimal wound healing, the wound bed should be clean and free of devitalised tissue. Dressings should not be adherent to the wound bed; otherwise, when these are removed or the dressings are changed, healing tissue will be removed with the dressing. Simple wound dressings such as paraffin-impregnated gauze are no longer routinely used in burns, and newer dressings that have a silicone surface such as Mepitel or Mepilex are better as they can be removed without disturbing the wound bed. In general, silver-based dressings such as Mepilex Ag are used in burn wounds as they have a direct antimicrobial activity.

Multidisciplinary Approach in Burn Management

A multidisciplinary approach to the treatment of burns is essential. A number of different teams bring specific expertise to the management of children with burns:

- **Allied health involvement is core to the management of paediatric burns**

Burns in children can have a significant impact on the child and family both physically and psychosocially and in the long and short term. Children with large burns have increased caloric requirements and often need additional supplements and feeds that can be guided by a **dietician**.

Occupational therapists and **physiotherapists** are important in the short and long term for mobility and scar management. Early mobilisation, particularly after large burns, is useful in preventing contractures from forming and also in reducing loss of muscle bulk. Early mobilisation once the graft has taken should be encouraged and facilitated by physiotherapists and occupational therapists.

Support can be provided to the child and the family by **social workers**, **indigenous liaison officers** and **psychologists**. This is particularly important for children with large burns who may require prolonged hospitalisation in a tertiary burn centre far away from home.

It is extremely important to ensure that patients with burns have appropriate analgesia during the acute phase of the injury and also for dressing changes and after any surgery. The involvement of our **anaesthetic** colleagues to facilitate this is an integral component in providing optimal care for the burn. Untreated pain from a burn can result in physiological derangement which impairs optimal healing and psychological distress from untreated pain can result in both short-term and longer-term problems for families.

Importantly, non-accidental injury should always be considered in children with atypical history or delayed presentation of burns. Where there is any suspicion, a child safety report and **social worker** involvement are mandatory.

Scar Management

Scar and contracture management is important both acutely and in the long term. Partial-thickness and full-thickness burns can form early contractures due to swelling. It is vitally important that these children have splinting from the beginning. When surgery is delayed, it is important to maintain joints in the correct functional position and prevent contractures from forming. Once a burn has been grafted, it is equally important to maintain an optimal position to prevent contractures and also to immobilise the graft to prevent graft loss from shearing forces.

Any burn that takes longer than 2 weeks to heal is at risk of healing with a hypertrophic scar. This is particularly true in patients with either very pale or very dark skin tones. The **Fitzpatrick scale** is a numerical classification for human skin colour, developed to estimate the response of different skin types to UV light. There are six types of skin tones described in the Fitzpatrick scale:

- *Type I*: Always burns, never tans, pale, freckles
- *Type II*: Usually burns, tans minimally
- *Type III*: Sometimes mild burn, tans uniformly (golden honey or olive skin tone)
- *Type IV*: Burns minimally, always tans well (moderate brown)
- *Type V*: Very rarely burns, tans easily (dark brown)
- *Type VI*: Never burns (deeply pigmented dark brown)

Patients with type I and type V–VI skin types are at greatest risk of hypertrophic scar formation. This is particularly problematic for Aboriginal and Torres Strait Islander patients in our population in North Queensland. Children are at higher risk of hypertrophic scar formation than adults. The mainstay of scar prevention is the use of pressure dressings that exert a constant, continual pressure on the wound as it heals. Pressure garments should be worn until the scar is mature (this usually takes from 6 to 18 months). It is often difficult to persuade children and their families of the importance of wearing these garments. They are custom-made to fit the injured area and need to be measured carefully to ensure an adequate fit. There is a need to change the garments as the child grows and also to replace the dressings if they become damaged or worn out. We depend heavily on the occupational therapists both in our unit and in surrounding units to help families manage pressure garments in the community.

Special Burns

Chemical burns

In children, caustic injuries represent an uncommon but serious problem. The common causative agents are household cleaning products which may be alkali (more common, produce liquefactive necrosis) or acidic (produce coagulative necrosis). Immediate first aid involves thorough irrigation of affected areas including inside of the mouth with water. It is important where possible to determine the contents of the chemical involved as some chemicals may also cause systemic toxicity. It can be difficult to assess the severity of burns in a young child, and endoscopic assessment is usually required. Oesophageal burns can result in acute ulceration or perforation and chronic stricture formation.

Electrical burns

Electrical injuries are divided into low voltage (<1000 V) and high voltage (>1000 V). Low-voltage burns typically occur at home and may be secondary to a child putting their fingers into a power socket, faulty cords or biting electrical cords. High-voltage burns are less common and may result from power lines or lightning strikes. All children with electrical burns should be examined for an entrance and exit wound, which are typically full-thickness burns. High-voltage injuries are associated with damage to the deep tissues, including muscle, which can be extensive and lead to rhabdomyolysis. An electrocardiogram (ECG) should be performed to assess for arrhythmias, and children with any abnormal findings require a period of telemetry. The typical appearances of an electrical burn on the hand of an infant can be seen in Figure 9.5.

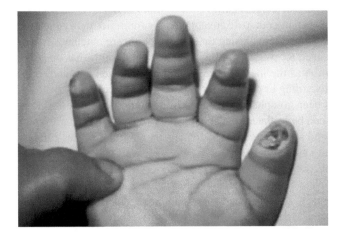

FIGURE 9.5   Full-thickness electrical burn.

Late Complications of Burns

Burns carry the risk of ongoing problems of burnt areas. It is important that families are told to reduce UV exposure to burnt tissue and donor sites. The psychological outcomes for families that have children who have suffered burn injuries are just starting to be appreciated. Where necessary, involvement of psychological support for children and their families can be very helpful in managing the trauma associated with a burn, particularly when they involve cosmetic deformities.

It is common for burnt areas and donor sites to become itchy following a burn. This is due to a combination of factors, but in particular, the lack of moisture in the damaged tissue is important. The regular application of non-scented simple moisturiser is often helpful in reducing itch and improving the character of a scar (reduced raised areas increase pliability and can improve pain).

Future Advances in Burn Management

The progress in the management of burns in children over the past 10 years has been astonishing. A number of advances have been made in terms of our early management of burns, as well as new technologies with dressings, matrix, improvements in the multidisciplinary management of cases and the use of allograft and tissue engineering to grow skin cells or extract skin cells into solution (Recell). Despite this, burn management is challenging and utilises a significant amount of resources. Our management in the future is likely to involve improving the morbidity from burns and, in particular, in improving outcomes from scarring. The use of fractional laser resurfacing of the skin using carbon dioxide lasers is showing much early promise in the management of troublesome scars by improving scar flexibility, appearance and helping with pain and itch. Other lasers such as pulsed dye lasers can also help with the appearance and redness in scars. We are actively exploring the use of CO_2 lasers in our patients with problematic scars following burns.

SUMMARY

Burns are a common injury in our patient group. **Most burns are preventable**, and future strategies for managing burns should always include prevention as the key message in reducing the burden of disease in our communities.

Once a burn has occurred, **a significant reduction in harm can be achieved by early, adequate and appropriate first aid**. Reaching out to disadvantaged communities with educational messaging surrounding, this is an important strategy in closing the gap in healthcare outcomes in disadvantaged groups such as ATSI families. The need for surgery for the management of burns has decreased dramatically over the past 15 years in Australia as the messages regarding burn prevention, and, in particular, the successful population education regarding first aid in burns have been successful.

Once first aid has been completed, then the child should be transferred to healthcare facility where appropriate treatment can be initiated. For the majority of cases, burns are superficial and will heal with appropriate dressings and adequate care. The management of these cases can be facilitated by local burn teams using telehealth to guide management.

A small number of cases need to be transferred to tertiary-level centres for further treatment. Surgery may be limited to simple wound debridement and application of dressings, but if the skin is extensively damaged, then skin-grafting may be necessary. The management of these injuries is best undertaken in specialist centres where a large multidisciplinary team work together to achieve the best outcomes for these patients. Careful management of the wounds and donor sites with appropriate dressings and thermoplastic splinting are usually sufficient to result in good outcomes for our patients.

A very small number of patients present with critical injuries from burns. These patients typically have a greater than 10% TBSA burn and can have associated polytrauma or other injuries that require paediatric intensive care support. The appropriate, timely and safe transfer of these patients after direct liaison with a burn specialist is key to attaining good outcomes in this small group of patients.

FURTHER READING

Butts CC, Holmes JH, Carter JE. Surgical escharotomy and decompressive therapies in burns. J Burn Care Res. 2020 February;41(2):263–9.

Cuttle L, Fear M, Wood FM, Kimble RM, Holland AJA. Management of non-severe burn wounds in children and adolescents: Optimising outcomes through all stages of the patient journey. Lancet Child Adolesc Health. 2022 April;6(4):269–78.

Cuttle L, Pearn J, McMillan JR, Kimble RM. A review of first aid treatments for burn injuries. Burns. 2009 September;35(6):768–75.

Fraser S, Grant J, Mackean T, Hunter K, Holland AJA, Clapham K, Teague WJ, Ivers RQ. Burn injury models of care: A review of quality and cultural safety for care of indigenous children. Burns. 2018 May;44(3):665–77.

Strobel AM, Fey R. Emergency care of pediatric burns. Emerg Med Clin North Am. 2018 May;36(2):441–58.

Zuccaro J, Ziolkowski N, Fish J. A systematic review of the effectiveness of laser therapy for hypertrophic burn scars. Clin Plast Surg. 2017 October;44(4):767–79.

Paediatric Urology

A Simplified Approach to Dealing with Urinary Tract Dilatation

10

Daniel Carroll

Paediatric urology is a distinct subspecialty of paediatric surgery specialising in the management of conditions of the genitourinary tract of boys and girls. Although this may sound as if it is quite a narrow area of practice, the incidence of congenital and acquired problems of the genitourinary tract is sufficiently high that paediatric urological problems account for roughly one-third of all referrals to paediatric surgical departments. A more detailed description of these problems is beyond the scope of this chapter, and here we will limit discussion to the most commonly encountered in clinical practice with particular reference to the difference and management difficulties of such problems in the context of remote and rural distribution of patients in a tropical environment. Areas covered in other chapters such as problems of the external genitalia (Chapter 13) are discussed in detail elsewhere.

ANTENATALLY DETECTED RENAL TRACT ANOMALIES

Abnormalities of the renal tract (now often termed congenital abnormalities of the kidney and urinary tract [CAKUT]) are one of the most commonly identified antenatal malformations. Over the past decade, with improvements in ultrasound scanning (USS) technology and operator experience, the incidence of CAKUT detected prenatally has risen from 1:200 to around 1:50 pregnancies. Routine USS is typically undertaken at 13 and 20 weeks of gestation in uncomplicated pregnancies. Dilatation of the collecting system, either the renal pelvis or distal ureter, accounts for the vast majority of cases. Most cases demonstrate only minor abnormalities, and treatment is largely conservative. As a guide, only around one in ten cases subsequently require surgical intervention. A number of factors can help predict those patients most likely to require surgical intervention or further investigations or management in infancy, and it is these patients and their families that benefit most from antenatal counselling by paediatric urologists and prenatal planning of postnatal patient management. This is particularly important for families who live in remote and rural areas as healthcare resources can often be more limited, and it may be difficult for families to access

DOI: 10.1201/9781003156659-10

127

these resources. It is important to consider that vulnerable patient groups such as Aboriginal and Torres Strait Islander (ATSI) patients and their families may require extra resources and support to achieve the best long-term outcomes.

CLASSIFICATION OF ANTENATAL HYDRONEPHROSIS (AHN)

Antenatal hydronephrosis (AHN) complicates between 1 and 5% of pregnancies and is the most commonly antenatally detected congenital abnormality. In 1993, the Society for Fetal Urology (SFU) proposed a grading system that provides a qualitative assessment of hydronephrosis on the basis of the antenatal appearance of the urinary tract. In particular, it examines the degree of pelviectasis and presence or absence of cortical or renal parenchymal thinning. This system stratifies patients into one of five groups, ranging from a score of 0 (normal) to group 4 (severe disease). This system has been criticised because of its limitation of high interobserver variability, particularly for patients in groups 2 and 3.

Other investigators have used a quantitative measurement of renal tract dilatation by measuring the anterior-to-posterior diameter (APD) of the renal pelvis on USS-acquired images in the transverse plane. Whilst it has the advantage of lesser interobserver variability, it is possible to be misled in kidneys that have a markedly abnormal collecting system with only minor changes in measured APD. Conversely, it is possible to overestimate risk for patients with a large extrarenal pelvis but normal collecting system if care is not taken to measure the APD in exactly the right position.

The SFU grade correlates well with the need for further urological treatment and interventions in childhood. Patients with grade 1 disease on this system have only a 2% chance of subsequently requiring surgical intervention in childhood, whilst those with SFU grade 4 have an almost 100% likelihood of subsequent surgical intervention. In 2009, the Canadian Urological and Paediatric Urological Association produced a useful guideline for the management of patients with antenatally diagnosed hydronephrosis on the basis of the SFU grade and measurement of APD which was updated in 2015. It is possible to stratify ANH on the basis of a quantitative measure of APD during fetal life into mild, moderate or severe disease.

TABLE 10.1   SFU classification of AHN on basis of renal morphology

SFU GRADING SYSTEM

- Grade 0 (normal)
    - No dilatation calyceal walls are apposed
- Grade 1 (mild)
    - Dilatation of the renal pelvis without calyceal dilatation
    - Dilatation of the extrarenal pelvis
    - No parenchymal atrophy
- Grade 2 (mild)
    - Dilatation of the renal pelvis and one or more major calyces
    - No parenchymal atrophy
- Grade 3 (moderate)
    - Dilatation of the renal pelvis and dilatation of all three major calyces
    - Blunting of fornices and flattening of papillae
- Grade 4 (severe)
    - Gross dilatation of the renal pelvis and calcyces
    - Renal atrophy (cortical thinning)

Severity of AHN by APD

The third component of renal tract abnormalities that should be considered prior to birth is the size of the fetal bladder. A useful determinant of megacystis is that the fetal bladder sagittal length should be no longer in millimetres than the gestational age + 2.

TABLE 10.2   Classification of AHN on basis of APD

DEGREE OF ANH	SECOND TRIMESTER APD (MM)	THIRD TRIMESTER APD (MM)
Mild	4 to <7	7 to <9
Moderate	7 to ≤ 10	9 to ≤ 15
Severe	>10	>15

There is a strong positive correlation between the degree of AHN and the presence of persistent or progressive disease.

TABLE 10.3   Correlation between antenatal findings and postnatal pathology

DEGREE OF ANH	REPORTED INCIDENCE (%)	INCIDENCE OF POSTNATAL PATHOLOGY (%)
Mild	57–88	12
Moderate	10–30	45
Severe	1.5–13	88

Given this strong association, it would seem reasonable to focus resources including antenatal counselling for those patients at highest risk of progression (i.e. patients with moderate and severe AHN) to allow for planning of perinatal management (geographical location of delivery, postnatal investigations, multidisciplinary team communication).

Postnatal Management of Patients with AHN

Whilst individualised care is the ideal situation, the following steps are usually important to consider.

Clinical Examination

A thorough and complete examination of a child with a known renal tract abnormality is essential. It is important to look for the following features as well as completing a more general examination:

- Palpable kidney
- Palpable bladder
- Stigmata of neural tube defects
- Normal introitus
- Normal external genitalia

Investigations

In patients with bilateral severe AHN or with a solitary kidney with AHN or abnormal renal echogenicity, a baseline creatinine should be performed after 48 h.

USS renal tract

Where possible, this should be delayed or repeated until 48 h after birth because relative oliguria in neonates may underestimate the degree of postnatal HN:

- Kidney length
- Kidney echogenicity/corticomedullary differentiation
- SFU grade HN
- Presence of hydroureteronephrosis (HUN)
- APD measurement
- Bladder volume/thickness/trabeculation/diverticula
- Look for signs of proximal urethral obstruction (keyhole sign)
- Where possible postvoid images should be acquired as well

Micturating cystourethrogram (MCUG)

This test is most useful in male infants suspected having bladder outlet obstruction. It often adds little to the management of other causes of AHN which can often resolve spontaneously and carries a small risk of introducing infection. This should be mitigated against by giving patients antibiotics before and after the procedure. It is often necessary for the paediatric urologist to catheterise the child for this procedure.

Radionucleotide studies (nuclear medicine)

These tests can be divided up into *static* and *dynamic* studies.

In dynamic studies, e.g., MAG3/DTPA radiolabelled studies use a tracer which is radiolabelled with technetium. This then allows for images to be captured afterwards, which give an estimation of differential renal function and the ability of the radiolabel to be cleared from the collecting system. It is important that this test is done in a standardised manner (the SFU described 'the well-tempered renogram' in 1992 stressing the importance of standardisation of techniques including ensuring that the patient is adequately hydrated, and the bladder is catheterised. The relatively poor uptake of tracer in the neonatal kidney limits this investigation's usefulness in children in the first month of life, and, where possible, the test should be deferred until reproducible and reliable images can be obtained (typically after 4 weeks of age). Administration of frusemide to determine the time to clear half of the tracer and the shape of the drainage curve after a diuretic challenge is essential, and so patients are either given this concomitantly with the radiolabelled tracer or a few minutes afterwards. In practice, the lack of standardisation of tests is not usually a problem clinically as long as the interpretation of the result is based upon a clear understanding of how the test was performed.

In static studies (DMSA scan), a radiolabelled tracer that is not eliminated is injected intravenously. The static nature of the study allows for a much clearer evaluation of the morphology of the kidney allowing for multiple images to be taken from different angles. This allows for a more accurate assessment of differential renal function and an appreciation of more subtle areas of photopenia that correspond to areas of relative nonfunction of the kidney. The acquisition of oblique views is particularly helpful in identifying small areas of renal scarring that most commonly arise in the upper and lower calyces of the kidney where the collecting ducts are crowded together, and intrarenal reflux is most likely to occur. This test is most typically performed later in childhood, often after suspected pyelonephritis to look for renal scarring, or to characterise differential function in duplex systems. It is most commonly used in the assessment of infants when seeking to confirm the presence of a multi-cystic dysplastic kidney. In this condition, the abnormal development of the renal tissue antenatally results in a completely non-functioning kidney (0% on differential function). These patients can often be managed conservatively in infancy.

Other tests in infancy

In selected infants, cystoscopy may be useful. Direct visualisation of the lower urinary tract can be helpful in identifying ectopic ureters, confirming the presence and offering treatment options for ureterocoeles, treating and diagnosing posterior urethral valves, primary non-refluxing megaureters (PNRMs) and vesicoureteric reflux (VUR). Although it usually offers the most information, it suffers from the disadvantage of requiring general anaesthesia and instrumentation of the urethra.

For patients with complex urinary abnormalities then MRU can offer excellent images when evaluating complex abnormalities. This is particularly useful in patients with other complex anatomical abnormalities (such as VACTERL anomalies and anorectal malformations). It is often possible to perform this study utilising a feed and wrap technique rather than anaesthesia in infants, and MR cross-sectional imaging has the added advantage of not requiring ionising radiation; however, in practice, images are often suboptimal without the use of general anaesthesia.

Continuous Antibiotic Prophylaxis (CAP)

In an attempt to improve the long-term outcomes for patients diagnosed with AHN, empirical continuous antibiotic prophylaxis has been the mainstay of conservative management for over 30 years. It is important to acknowledge that whilst the use of CAP is accepted and probably of benefit for young children (<2 years of age) with moderate and severe hydronephrosis, the evidence base supporting its use remains weak. There is probably insufficient evidence at this stage to support its use in patients with only mild- or low-grade AHN as a routine. In our practice, patients returning to remote and isolated areas with limited access to healthcare resources can be at significant risk if they develop urosepsis and out of an abundance of caution selected patients are often commenced on continuous antibiotic prophylaxis after consultation with the family. The SFU consensus statement on CAP in 2010 only recommends CAP for patients with high-grade hydronephrosis and proven VUR. For every seven patients with high-grade hydronephrosis treated with CAP, we will prevent one episode of urinary tract infection (UTI). In those patients with megaureters, 34% have a febrile UTI in the first 6 months of life. Male patients with significant upper tract anomalies (e.g. megaureters/PUV) almost certainly accrue significant protection from longer-term renal damage from neonatal circumcision, and this should be discussed with families (ideally antenatally) to allow them to make a timely, informed decision regarding circumcision.

Commonly used antimicrobials used for CAP include amoxicillin, cephalexin and trimethoprim. Trimethoprim sulfamethoxazole (Bactrim) and nitrofurantoin should be avoided in the neonate because of the respective risks of kernicterus and haemolytic anaemia.

A Simplified Approach to the Management of Antenatal Hydronephrosis

Although many excellent algorithms exist for the management of patients with AHN, I have found it useful to simplify this to ensure patients do not get under- or over-investigated. Patients with a solitary kidney and another abnormality of the renal tract or those with bilateral hydronephrosis or kidney disease as well as those patients with severe unilateral disease should, where possible, be reviewed antenatally by a paediatric urologist. This not only allows for planning of investigations and treatment immediately after delivery but also allows the surgical team to build rapport with the family.

After birth, those at highest risk of requiring intervention should have a USS once the period of postnatal relative oliguria has resolved (usually after 48 h following delivery). Practically this means that it may be necessary to remain in hospital until assessments by the paediatric and or neonatal team have appropriately assessed the baby. For the smaller group of patients who have been demonstrated to have severe unilateral disease or with bilateral renal disease should be referred to paediatric urology for ongoing management. This may include the institution of CAP and require further investigations prior to discharge (e.g. MCUG) dependent upon the clinical progress and the results of the early USS. Most patients with moderate or severe disease require a minimum 3-monthly USS and regular clinical reviews as well as parent education and liaison with local healthcare providers (GPs/paediatricians) as to the signs and symptoms of renal tract obstruction and or urosepsis and renal insufficiency. It is usual for these patients to be commenced on appropriate CAP as discussed earlier.

Dilatation of the collecting system and ureters

With improvements in antenatal care and scanning technology around nine out of ten clinically significant urinary tract abnormalities are detected during pregnancy. If a child presents with hydronephrosis or HUN after birth, then it is usually following investigation with renal tract ultrasonography as a consequence of UTI or symptomatic renal disease (loin pain/haematuria etc.). It is increasingly common for children to present to clinic for advice and management of abnormal renal tract USS findings after having undergone USS as a component of generalised investigations (incidental finding). The natural history of asymptomatic renal tract abnormalities is poorly understood.

USS is an excellent modality for examining the structure of the kidney and the collecting systems. Hydronephrosis and HUN occur for two main reasons. The first is due to an impairment of drainage of the urinary tract (loosely termed obstruction); the second is because of abnormalities of reflux from the bladder into the collecting system (VUR). It is not possible to distinguish between these two separate entities on the basis of USS alone, but serial or dynamic USS examinations can allow the astute clinician to infer that one of these two causes is more likely than the other. Of particular value in this regard is the acquisition of post-voiding images, which often show significant improvement of HUN with an empty bladder. Sometimes it is possible to capture images showing progressive dilatation of the ureters during voiding suggesting VUR is responsible for the HUN. For the majority of patients with low grade, asymptomatic renal tract dilatation serial monitoring with USS is sufficient. For patients with severe, bilateral or progressive renal tract dilatation, further investigations are warranted (see Figure 10.4).

Impairment of flow in the urinary tract

If drainage of the collecting system is impaired, it is most commonly due to 'obstruction' at one of two anatomical locations. For patients with hydronephrosis, we should consider whether there is pelvi-ureteric junction dysfunction (previously termed PUJO). For patients with HUN, we need to consider whether this is due to impairment of flow lower down the collecting system (most commonly at the vesico-ureteric junction). When there is a dilated ureter visible on the USS, then this is termed a PNRM. In some instances, a combination of PUJO and VUR exists (VUR complicates up to 10% of all cases of PUJO). For the purposes of simplicity, we will subdivide management into these two major separate groups.

PUJ dysfunction

Incidence: 1:1500

Presentation: Typically presents antenatally with AHN (90%) can present with UTI or symptoms (e.g. loin pain, haematuria) a number present incidentally with a mass or abnormal USS findings.

Findings: Usually there is progressive hydronephrosis with often moderate or severe disease on USS. The diagnosis is usually confirmed using dynamic radionucleotide imaging (MAG3 or DTPA scan). (An example of a patient with PUJO can be seen in Figures 10.1 and 10.2.)

Natural history: Some patients with mild or moderate disease improve throughout childhood, although at least 10% who initially show improvement may subsequently exhibit progressive disease later in childhood. This is often due to the presence of 'crossing vessels' where the abnormal anatomical arrangement of the renal vessels as the ureter crosses over them has a potential to cause kinking of the ureter. These patients most commonly present with symptoms of loin pain in adolescence.

Investigations: Ultrasonography of the renal tract is cheap, painless and readily available even in remote and rural locations. As such, it is an ideal modality to monitor disease progress. It is

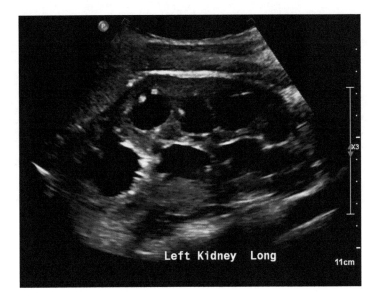

FIGURE 10.1   Ultrasound showing left hydronephrosis.

generally accepted that even in asymptomatic patients, the presence of an anterior-posterior diameter (APD) of the pelvi-ureteric junction of >30 mm is sufficient to warrant further investigation. For those patients with an APD >35 mm then the requirement for operative intervention approaches 100%. Once surgery is being considered, it is usual to arrange for dynamic radionucleotide imaging of the renal tract (either a MAG3 or DTPA scan) dependent upon local availability and preference. It is important to remember that these scans are slightly different, and DTPA scans reflect glomerular filtration and so rely on glomerular filtration rate (GFR) and are unreliable and difficult to interpret in neonates who have a low GFR. These tests, when performed well, provide an excellent measure of renal drainage and differential function. A drop in function to <40% or a clearly obstructed drainage curve are indications for surgical intervention.

Surgery: For those patients requiring surgery then, it is possible to perform either an open or laparosopic dismembered Anderson–Hynes pyeloplasty. It is my practice to perform retrograde pyelography first to exclude distal ureteric obstruction which can become evident after fixing an obstructed PUJ. This can occur in up to 10% of patients with PUJ dysfunction. This operation has a high success rate with a low complication rate and essentially removes the non-functioning PUJ, and the renal pelvis is then tailored and anastomosed to the distal ureter. In younger children, the technical demands of performing the procedure usually dictate an open approach or a transperitoneal laparoscopic approach.

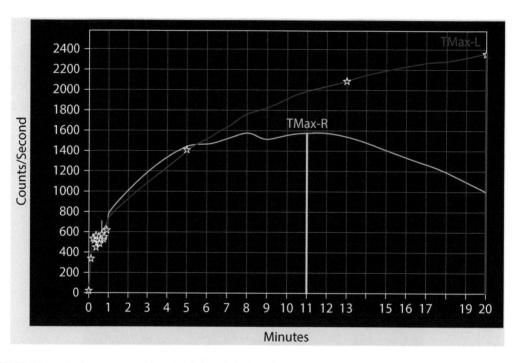

FIGURE 10.2   Drainage curves showing left PUJ dysfunction.

Primary non-refluxing megaureter (PNRM)

Vesicoureteric junction dysfunction or obstruction (VUJO) can result in HUN (a dilatation of the ureter and renal pelvis/collecting system). More recently, many clinicians also choose to term this condition a PNRM. Historically, treatment was typically surgical by ureteric reimplantation. Advances in our understanding of the natural history of this condition over the last 40 years have led to the adoption of a more conservative approach, with a combination of medical treatment to prevent infection (CAP) combined with careful surveillance to watch for progression of disease and minimally invasive approaches for those with progressive or symptomatic disease. Patients with a progressive megaureter or pyonephrosis should be considered for surgery, and an increasing number of surgical options are available. In general, younger children can be managed with less invasive strategies, which may serve as a temporising measure. Evidence of severe HUN should prompt the surgeon to investigate further with dynamic nucleotide imaging (e.g. MAG3 scan). A loss of function or episodes of pyonephrosis are relative indications for surgical intervention. A progressive dilatation of the retrovesical ureter to >2.0 cm is usually associated with a need for surgical intervention.

Surgery for PNRM
For children under the age of 2 years, bladder surgery is often complicated by longer-term bladder dysfunction. It is, therefore, my practice wherever possible to adopt a more conservative strategy in younger patients. Cystoscopy and endoscopic placement of a soft double J stent across the vesicoureteric junction is often successful as a temporising measure. There is evidence to suggest that this may be sufficient alone to treat PNRM in a substantial number of patients. It is important to carefully manage young children with stents in situ to make sure the stent does not migrate or cause other problems, and they should be changed regularly in infants. In patients with complex PNRM (those with repeated pyonephrosis, bilateral disease or reduced renal function demonstrable on radionucleotide imaging), then ureteric reimplantation may be necessary. Certainly, this is an effective and reliable operation.

Vesicoureteric reflux

Although there are other causes of 'obstruction', such as uterine polyps and renal stones, the majority of patients with HUN or HN without demonstrable 'obstruction' suffer from VUR. Prior to the 1980s, this was the principal cause of renal failure in childhood and as such was the focus of much surgical endeavour in an attempt to alter the natural history of this condition. Historically, patients with VUR underwent ureteric reimplantation in childhood. Two major subsequent studies were undertaken to look at the role of CAP in the management of VUR, and both reported independently that similar (if not better) patient outcomes could be achieved by adopting a conservative strategy with CAP compared to surgical interventions. These findings led to a huge paradigm shift away from the surgical treatment of VUR.

A few years after this, paediatric urologists in Dublin (P Puri and B O'Donnell) proposed a novel surgical therapy for the treatment of VUR by injecting inert substances into the vesicoureteric junction to improve VUR. This 'STING' procedure (sub-ureteric injection) proved to be very successful and subsequent refinements to the technique and improvement in the materials used for injection have led to a significant reduction in the number of children undergoing open surgery for the treatment of VUR. For those patients with complex or progressive VUR, ureteric reimplantation remains an excellent surgical therapy, with good long-term outcomes and low complication rates.

The majority of patients with high-grade VUR present prenatally, with HUN detected antenatally. A smaller number of patients, often with lower grade VUR, present later in childhood with UTIs. It is important for the clinician to differentiate between primary and secondary VURs. In primary VUR, the abnormal or ectopic position of the ureteric orifice in relation to the trigone results in an inadequate intravesical tunnel of ureter within the bladder wall. This anatomical abnormality results in failure of the normal 'flap valve' mechanism which ordinarily prevents reflux of urine from the bladder back into the distal ureter during micturition. The ectopic positioning of the ureter is usually associated with primary VUR. In this condition, the pressures within the bladder are normal both at rest and during voiding, and so reflux occurs due to a failure of the normally passive mechanism of distal ureteric closure during micturition. When urine refluxes into the ureter during voiding, there is an incomplete elimination of urine from the bladder, as urine passes backwards into the ureter and collecting system, once micturition is complete the urine then passively drains into the bladder leaving a 'pseudoresidual'. This incomplete emptying of urine provides a potential reservoir of infection and is thought to be the contributing factor towards the increased risk of UTIs in children with VUR. Treatment of this patient group with CAP (and consideration of circumcision in male infants) results in reduced bacterial load and this probably accounts for their effectiveness in preventing UTIs in this group of patients. In secondary VUR, the reflux of urine into the ureters is caused by an abnormally high pressure at various stages during filling and emptying of the bladder. It is important to consider this as a cause for reflux as untreated bladder outlet obstruction, and a high-pressure system can often lead to a subsequent decline in renal function, and there is a longer-term risk of renal insufficiency. The commonest cause of secondary VUR is detrusor overactivity (DO). This may be related to chronic inflammation of the bladder or learned behaviours during toilet training (e.g. detrusor sphincter dyssynergia [DSD]). For male patients, it is important to consider the possibility of a high-pressure bladder with bladder outlet obstruction resulting from a rare congenital disorder called posterior urethral valves.

Posterior urethral valves

The most serious potential cause of AHN in male infants is posterior urethral valves. Posterior urethral valves (PUV) are obstructive abnormal leaflets of tissue in the posterior urethra causing an obstruction. Previously, they were categorised into three categories by Hugh Hampton Young, but current evidence suggests that they may more accurately be described as a congenital obstructing posterior urethral membrane (COPUM).

Introduction

Posterior urethral valves have a reported incidence of 1:5000 live male births. Up to 50% of patients progress to end-stage renal disease during childhood. Improvements in antenatal diagnosis and early intervention and management have largely failed to deliver on improving outcomes for end stage renal disease (ESRD), and it must be presumed that much of the renal damage happens prior to birth (or diagnosis).

Treatment/Management Options

There are no validated criteria for antenatal intervention, although vesico-amniotic shunting may improve bladder function. Antenatal counselling is useful for families and for neonatal and paediatric urology teams to plan management after delivery. Antenatal intervention is associated with significant morbidity and mortality. In general, fetal surgery is not routinely recommended outside the context of clinical trials.

Postnatal Management

There is a wide variety of clinical presentations after delivery. Some patients have significant oligohydramnios and subsequent pulmonary hypoplasia and moulding deformities. The initial management is dictated by the neonatal team and is supportive. It may be necessary to seek advice and help from the paediatric nephrologist to optimise and support renal function and manage electrolyte imbalances.

Following stabilisation of the infant a catheter is inserted, often with the help of a paediatric urologist as insertion can be difficult due to the abnormal angulation of the posterior urethra. Diagnosis is usually confirmed with an MCUG (being careful to ensure that the baby is well prior to the procedure, and that appropriate antibiotic coverage is provided) (see Figure 10.3).

Cystoscopic valve ablation is performed once the baby is well. VUR is common, and prophylactic antibiotics should be continued. In the case of premature infants, cystoscopic ablation is often not possible, and a vesicostomy may be required. A simplified algorithm for the management of uncomplicated renal tract abnormalities in children is laid out in Figure 10.4.

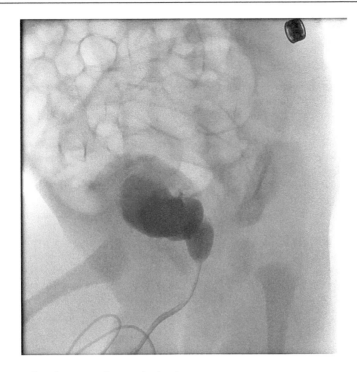

FIGURE 10.3   MCUG showing posterior urethral valves.

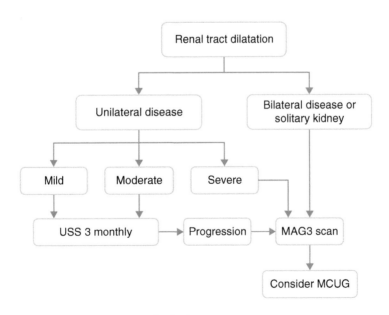

FIGURE 10.4   MCUG showing posterior urethral valves.

FURTHER READING

Al Aaraj MS, Badreldin AM. Ureteropelvic junction obstruction. In: StatPearls [Internet]. Treasure Island (FL): StatPearls Publishing; 2022 January [Updated 11 July 2022].

Deshpande AV. Current strategies to predict and manage sequelae of posterior urethral valves in children. Pediatr Nephrol. 2018 October;33(10):1651–61.

Farrugia MK, Hitchcock R, Radford A, Burki T, Robb A, Murphy F. British association of paediatric urologists. British association of paediatric urologists consensus statement on the management of the primary obstructive megaureter. J Pediatr Urol. 2014 February;10(1):26–33.

Läckgren G, Cooper CS, Neveus T, Kirsch AJ. Management of vesicoureteral reflux: What have we learned over the last 20 years? Front Pediatr. 2021 March;9:650326.

Lissauer D, Morris RK, Kilby MD. Fetal lower urinary tract obstruction. Semin Fetal Neonatal Med. 2007 December;12(6):464–70.

Nguyen HT, Benson CB, Bromley B, Campbell JB, Chow J, Coleman B, Cooper C, Crino J, Darge K, Herndon CD, Odibo AO, Somers MJ, Stein DR. Multidisciplinary consensus on the classification of prenatal and postnatal urinary tract dilation (UTD classification system). J Pediatr Urol. 2014 December;10(6):982–98.

Okarska-Napierała M, Wasilewska A, Kuchar E. Urinary tract infection in children: Diagnosis, treatment, imaging – Comparison of current guidelines. J Pediatr Urol. 2017 December;13(6):567–73.

Thoracic Surgery in Children

11

Kyle Crowley and Daniel Carroll

INTRODUCTION

A number of important conditions that involve the chest are commonplace in paediatric surgical practice. In general, these can be subdivided up into congenital and acquired abnormalities. In tropical areas, the incidence and presentation of patients with congenital abnormalities of the chest are similar to that seen in other geographical locations, but there is a marked difference in the presentation of acquired thoracic pathologies.

The thorax is the area marked superiorly by the first ribs and T1 vertebrae, and inferiorly by the diaphragm. It is enclosed by the ribcage and thoracic vertebra and includes the anterior and posterior chest walls. Contained within the thoracic cavity are the lungs, heart, and great vessels. Paediatric surgeons are mostly involved in the management of lesions that involve the chest wall, breast, and the lungs and oesophagus as operations involving the heart and great vessels are usually performed by subspecialist paediatric cardiac surgical services. For the purposes of this chapter, we will consider pathology from the outside of the chest working inwards commencing with pathologies involving the breast.

BREAST PATHOLOGIES

In the paediatric population, conditions of the breast are uncommon and typically benign or associated with normal breast development. A few conditions do require treatment, while most can be treated conservatively.

The breast undergoes two developmental stages, first during fetal development and a second during adolescence. The first stage occurs at between weeks 5 and 6 of fetal life with normal breast buds developing at the fourth intercostal space. The second stage, thelarche, occurs in response to oestrogen and progesterone leading to the development of the breast buds in females.

Galactorrhoea

Galactorrhoea or 'Witch's Milk' is a result of excess maternal hormones across the placenta during development resulting in hyperplasia of breast tissue and milk production. This occurs in about 5% of neonates

DOI: 10.1201/9781003156659-11

and occurs in either sex. The majority of cases resolve within a week when left alone, but the condition may persist for up to 2 months. Manipulation or attempting to express the milk may prolong the condition and potentially introduce bacteria that may lead to neonatal mastitis. In rare cases, oral oestrogen may be required to halt milk production.

Neonatal Mastitis

Mastitis is infection of breast tissue, typically occurring in the first few weeks of life classically in term neonates. It affects females twice as often as males. The most common causative organisms in the neonatal population are *Staphylococcus aureus*, followed by gram-negative enteric organisms, anaerobes, and Group B *Streptococcus*.

Mastitis is most commonly a localized infection rarely leading to generalized symptoms and systemic infection. Complete examination should be done to assess for the formation of an abscess. First-line treatment is antibiotics with appropriate coverage for *S. aureus*. If drainage of an abscess is required, aspiration or peri-areolar drainage is the preferred method to prevent reduced breast bud development and scarring, which can lead to uneven breast growth as an adolescent.

Precocious Puberty

Puberty is the transitional stage of development in childhood with rapid growth and development of secondary sexual characteristics. This occurs as a result of the maturation of the hypothalamic-pituitary-gonadal (HPG) axis. Activation of the HPG axis leads to stimulation and activation of hormones leading to testosterone release in males and oestradiol in females. This typically occurs in females between 8 and 13 years of age, and males between 9 and 14 years of age.

The development of secondary sexual characteristics in females before 8 years of age and males before 9 years of age is termed **precocious puberty**. This is a rare condition occurring more commonly in females than males.

Precocious puberty is broken into central and peripheral causes:

Central precocious puberty (CPP) is usually the result of earlier maturation and activation of the HPG axis. This tends to be idiopathic in females, but usually there is an underlying pathology in males. The most common causes include central nervous system tumours (hypothalamic hamartoma), CNS injury, syndromes (NF1), environmental, or genetics.

Peripheral precocious puberty (PPP) is the development of secondary sexual characteristics, independent of gonadotropin-releasing hormone (GnRH) pulsatile release, due to endogenous/exogenous sources of sex steroids. PPP is less common than CPP with causes, including congenital adrenal hyperplasia, gonadal tumours, adrenal tumours, and exogenous exposure to steroids.

The decision to treat in CPP is dependent on age and how rapidly puberty is progressing in the child. In PPP, treatment is directed at eliminating the source of the excess sex steroid.

Work-up is needed to help differentiate precocious puberty from benign forms of puberty, including premature thelarche, the premature development of breast tissue either unilaterally or bilaterally. This typically occurs between 12 and 24 months of age with no other associated pubertal changes. This requires frequent clinical follow-up to assure bilateral breast develop evenly, which may take 3–12 months to occur after diagnosis.

Adolescent Breast Conditions

There are a multitude of breast conditions in adolescent females that are commonly underexpressed as a concern in this population. Conditions can be broken into congenital/developmental, benign mass/tumours, malignant lesions, and other lesions, including infections and dermatological conditions:

- **Congenital and developmental** conditions include polythelia (supernumerary nipples), inverted nipples, athelia (absence of nipple), polymastia (supernumerary breast), and amastia. Treatment is usually cosmetic in nature to prevent body dysmorphic disorder.
- **Benign breast lesions** are most commonly fibroadenoma, accounting for 70–95% of biopsied lesions in this age. Biopsies should be avoided in the paediatric group to prevent breast tissue removal, which could result in asymmetrical breast development. These are oestrogen-sensitive and may or may not change with the menstrual cycle. In cases where the lesion is >5 cm (giant/juvenile fibroadenoma), excision may be warranted if it is fast growing, as the fibroadenoma may replace normal breast tissue. Discrete lesions in males and postpubertal females should almost always be removed.
- Cystosarcoma phyllodes is the most common **malignant breast tumour** in adolescent females but can often be benign. They should be evaluated with a 'triple test' of clinical history/examination, ultrasound, and non-excisional biopsy.
- **Adolescent mastitis** resembles that seen in adults and is managed similarly. Risk factors in adolescents include trauma (including plucking of hairs from nipple), lactation, duct obstruction, and immunocompromised status. Antibiotics are the treatment of choice. If an abscess has formed, percutaneous drainage is the preferred method with serial drainage until resolved. Incision and drainage should be reserved for abscesses >5 cm or abscesses that recur despite percutaneous drainage. *S. aureus* is the causative organism in an overwhelming majority of cases.

Gynaecomastia

Gynaecomastia is benign hyperplasia of glandular breast tissue. It can be physiological or pathological. Physiological gynaecomastia has a trimodal age distribution with peaks in newborns, adolescents, and men >50 years old. Sixty to ninety per cent of newborns are estimated to have gynaecomastia (neonatal mastauxe) as a result of maternal oestrogens which resolve within a few weeks of birth in a vast majority of cases. The second peak occurs in males between 10 and 19 years old with an estimated prevalence up to 69%. The cause for physiological gynaecomastia in adolescence is unclear. Studies evaluating oestrogen levels in adolescent gynaecomastia show normal levels in the majority of cases.

Pathological gynaecomastia can be associated with certain medical conditions, medication use, or substance abuse. If adolescent gynaecomastia hasn't resolved within 2 years of onset or 17 years of age, further investigation is warranted.

Common medical causes include primary/secondary hypogonadism, tumours, and malnutrition/disorders of impaired absorption. Medications/substances associated with gynaecomastia include metronidazole, omeprazole, marijuana, anabolic steroids, diazepam, alcohol, and metoclopramide. Treatment is aimed at treating the medical cause/ceasing the offending agent. In idiopathic causes with no other source found, treatment can be done with testosterone/oestrogen receptor modifying agents, or via surgery to improve cosmetic result.

CHEST WALL DEFORMITIES

Chest wall deformities (CWDs) are a congenital disease that can be an isolated condition, associated with other anomalies, or as part of a genetic syndrome. These conditions are often evident from birth. They are classified into five types according to the origin of the anomaly: cartilaginous, costal, chondro-costal, sternal, and clavicle-scapular (Table 11.1).

Type I: Cartilaginous Deformities

Pectus excavatum (**PE**) or 'funnel chest' is the most common thoracic malformation accounting for approximately 90% of CWDs. It is a concave recession in the chest wall due to malformation of the cartilaginous sternocostal joints leading to sternal protrusion with a reduced anteroposterior (AP) diameter of the thorax. It has a male predominance with a male to female ratio of 5:1. Commonly it is an isolated congenital condition that is identifiable at birth but commonly not picked up until the child is older. In situations where PE appears to develop later, approximately 15% of cases, it is more commonly associated with conditions of connective tissue development, including Marfans syndrome, Ehlers–Danlos syndrome, and osteogenesis imperfecta.

There is a strong familial association with up to 40% of cases having a family member also with PE. The deformity can be symmetrical or asymmetrical ranging from severe forms with a deep canal seeming to reach all the way to the vertebral column, to being barely noticeable with very little deformity.

Patients commonly are tall and thin, with joint laxity. There is an association with scoliosis or kypho-scoliosis in 15–50% of cases, but this rarely requires treatment. There is a rare association with cardiac anomalies, with mitral valve prolapse the most common associated anomaly. In some instances, in neonates with diaphragmatic hernia or respiratory obstruction, PE may resolve completely during infancy. Patients may complain of shortness of breath with exertion in severe cases.

When assessing the patient to determine if treatment is required, the gold standard is to perform a CT in order to assess the anatomy and calculate a Haller index score (Figure 11.1). The Haller index score is used to determine the sternal depression severity. A score on the Haller index greater than 3.25 is considered a severe defect requiring treatment. Additionally, pulmonary function tests and a thorough cardiac assessment must also be undertaken prior to surgical correction.

$$HI = \frac{\textit{Transverse diameter of inside ribcage}}{\textit{AP diameter between vertebrae and sternum}}$$

Timing of surgical correction is debated with good results seen in adult patients; however, generally there is an acceptance for correction in 9–15 years of age is a good age to consider surgery. Currently, the most widely performed surgical technique is the Nuss procedure in which a retrosternal metallic rod is bent

TABLE 11.1   Acastello classification of chest wall deformities

Type I: Cartilaginous	Pectus excavatum
	Pectus carinatum
Type II: Costal	Jeune syndrome
Type III: Chondro-costal	Poland syndrome
Type IV: Sternal	Sternal cleft
Type V: Clavicle-scapular	Clavicular
	Scapular combined

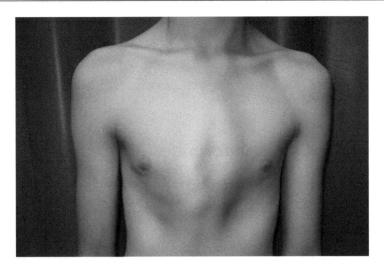

FIGURE 11.1 Pectus carinatum.

and rotated 180 degrees to instantly correct the deformity. The bar is removed a few years later after stabilization of the sternum. In rare severe cases, an open procedure is performed in which the sternum is mobilized, and costal cartilages divided to correct the deformity, then correct positioning maintained by steel struts behind the sternum.

Pectus carinatum (PC) or 'Pigeon Chest' is the protrusion of the sternum and costo-chondral cartilage – an example of a male child with PC can be seen in Figure 11.1. It is the second most common CWD, estimated to be four to five times less frequent than PE with a strong male predominance. The aetiology for PC is the same as that proposed for PE, but with protrusion of the ribs. It tends to present later around the time of puberty. A significant number of cases are familial in nature with a 25–30% positive family history. There are usually no associated cardiac abnormalities, but pulmonary symptoms are attributed to a fixed chest wall. In cases of impairment of superior limb movement, lung herniation, and flail chest, surgical repair is recommended. Presurgical work-up for patients with PC is similar to that of PE. There is no definitive cut-off for the Haller score, but a score of 1.9 is associated with dyspnea. Psychological effects in PC can be more significant than that of PE and are a fundamental indication for surgical correction.

PC is broken into Type 1 and Type 2 based on localization and symmetry. Type 1 or chondrogladiolar is the more frequent form with the protrusion occurring at the inferior/mid-sternum and more commonly symmetric compared to Type 2. Type 2 or chondromanubrial is at the superior aspect of the sternum due to premature fusion and ossification of the manubrio-sternal joint. There is commonly an associated inferior PE. The sternum on radiograph is 'S' shaped.

Surgically, Type 1 and Type 2 PC are approached differently. Type 2 requires an open repair with osteotomy of the sternal plate. Less invasive procedures have been proposed for Type 1 with good results, including: orthotic bracing/intrathoracic compression during puberty, thoracoscopic cartilage resection, and thoracoscopic complete cartilage resection with perichondrium preservation.

Type II: Costal Deformities

Costal defects are broken into non-syndromic and syndromic malformations. In non-syndromic costal, cartilage is malformed resulting in unilateral or bilateral depression of the thoracic wall. Treatment for non-syndromic form is via cartilage excision.

Jeune syndrome/asphyxiating thoracic dystrophy is autosomal recessive with an estimated prevalence of 1/100,000 to 1/30,000 live births. Jeune syndrome is described by multiple bone abnormalities, with the most severe being a narrow thorax with reduced lung capacity causing respiratory distress commonly resulting in death during infancy. It is subdivided into severe variant and mild variant with the severe variant making up ~70% of cases and typically resulting in death during infancy due to the small size of the thorax. The mild variant makes up 30% of cases and is manageable, eventual death may occur due to renal or hepatic dysfunction. Mild variants can be managed conservatively, while traditionally surgery was done via open sternotomy with poor results. Newer techniques include an expandable prosthetic titanium ribs, which has shown better results.

Type III: Chondro-Costal Deformities

Poland syndrome (PS) is a condition of absence or hypoplasia of pectoralis major along with ipsilateral deformities of the chest wall, breast, and upper limb. It occurs in an estimated 1 per 30,000 live births with male to female predominance of 2:1. Two-thirds of cases are described as being right sided and there are only rare reports of PS being bilateral.

The hypothesized cause of PS is disruption of subclavian and vertebral arteries during embryological development causing malformations in the corresponding supply areas. A lethal gene has been proposed as the origin of the anomaly, with a mosaic form leading to survival. PS has extreme variability in phenotype which ranges from mild sternal deformity without limb defect (Poland sequence) not picked up until childhood, to agenesis of ribs causing lung herniation and paradoxical chest movements. Surgical correction is indicated in psychosocial and chest wall/functional impairment. Surgery is recommended in adolescence after puberty with the aims of surgery being improvement of chest wall symmetry, anterior axillary fold creation, and hand reconstruction if required. The reconstruction is performed in multiple stages with stage 1 aim being skeletal reconstruction and stage 2 being thoracic soft tissue reconstruction. Hand defects are commonly repaired within 18–24 months of life.

Type IV: Sternal

Sternal cleft (SC) is a result of failure of the sternal valves fusion process during embryology. They make up 0.15% of CWDs with an estimated female predominance of 2:1. A majority is idiopathic but can be associated with syndromes, including PHACES syndrome and chromosome 22 syndromes. Inferior SC is usually syndromic with superior cleft being an isolated deformity. Deformities are classified as four types (Table 11.2). Consensus is for repair of SC to take place during the first months of life to re-establish bony protection of the mediastinum and allow normal growth of the thoracic cage.

Type V: Clavicle-Scapular Deformities

These deformities are managed by orthopaedic surgeons and outside the scope of this book.

TABLE 11.2 Shamberger and Welch classifications for sternal clefts

Sternal cleft	Malformation of thoracic wall due to deficient midline fusion.
Thoracic ectopia cordis	Heart is ectopic and not covered by skin with hypoplastic thoracic cavity. Few reported cases of survival.
Cervical ectopia cordis	Cranial heart sometimes fused to mouth with associated craniofacial anomalies. Poor prognosis.
Thoraco-abdominal ectopia cordis	Heart covered by thin membrane with inferior sternal defect, with heart located in lower thorax or abdomen. Post-surgical prognosis positive.

PULMONARY INFECTIONS

The diagnosis and management of pulmonary infections are similar between adults and children; however, extra considerations must be made in the paediatric population. Airways are smaller in the paediatric population increasing the risk for secretions and oedema to cause obstruction. In infancy, there is a weak cough reflex that is poor at clearance of mucus and exudate. Obstruction could potentiate infection and allow lobar collapse. In neonates, hypoxia can set in early causing increased respiratory effort and lead to respiratory failure. Changes in intrathoracic pressure are poorly tolerated and may lead to respiratory failure, especially with pre-existing lung disease.

In the majority of cases, surgical procedures to treat conditions of the pleura or lungs in the paediatric patient are either via resection of respiratory tissue or via pleural drainage. It is uncommon to have to intervene surgically as the majority of infective processes are managed conservatively and surgery is reserved for those with complex disease or failure of medical management.

Pneumonia

Pneumonia is an infection of the lower respiratory tract most commonly caused by viruses. Bacterial pneumonia is typically a secondary infection following viral pneumonia. World-wide pneumonia is the cause of 16% of deaths in children under 5 years old. In tropical regions, that number increases to 23% of child deaths. Pneumonia shows increased transmission in tropical climates during the rainy season. The most common causative bacteria in the Tropics are:

- *Streptococcus pneumoniae*
- *Klebsiella pneumoniae*
- *S. aureus*

Other causes seen almost exclusively in tropical areas are *Mycobacterium tuberculosis*, melioidosis (*Burkholderia pseudomallei*), and leptospirosis. Diagnosis with radiograph and sputum cultures helps direct therapy. Cases of bacterial pneumonia should be treated with antibiotics directed towards the most common causative organism and adjusted following culture. In most cases, pneumonias will resolve with antibiotics.

In rare cases, they may progress to empyema.

Empyema

Empyema thoracis is an uncommon complication of pneumonia typically resulting from a parapneumonic effusion, which turns into pus in the pleural space. The reported rate of childhood empyema from pneumonia in Australia is 0.7%. Mortality rates from empyema are low, but there is significant morbidity as a result of empyema. Prevalence of empyema continues to rise, including in tropical regions, with a disproportionately higher incidence rate amongst patients of Aboriginal and Torres Strait Islander (ATSI) background.

In Tropical Australia, the most common isolated organisms are non-multiresistant methicillin-resistant *S. aureus* in patients of ATSI background, while *S. pneumoniae* is the most commonly isolated organism in non-ATSI children. These organisms along with *Haemophilus influenzae*, *Mycoplasma pneumoniae*, and *Pseudomonas aeruginosa* are also the most common organisms worldwide.

TABLE 11.3 Stages of empyema

Pleural effusion	Fluid collection in pleural space as result of imbalance in lymphatic system. Vasculature becomes more permeable allowing inflammatory cells and bacteria in and form infection.
Exudative	Exudate low in cellular count accumulates in pleural space.
Fibrinopurulent	Presence of frank pus with an increase in white cells.
Organized	Formation of a thick peel and potential lung entrapment with very thick exudate and heavy sediment.

The typical clinical picture is that of a child presenting with symptoms of pneumonia that is more unwell than would be expected, often with pleuritic chest pain and reduced chest expansion. Reduced or absent breath sounds and dullness to percussion may be seen on examination with an evident effusion on chest radiography. Alternatively, it may be suspected in a child with known pneumonia who is not improving after 48 hours of antibiotics with persisting fevers.

Typical investigations in cases of suspected empyema include a plain chest radiography to identify a pleural effusion, most commonly unilateral in nature (Table 11.3). Ultrasound is the imaging modality of choice in pneumonia complicated by a parapneumonic effusion. In skilled hands, it is possible to distinguish between a simple pleural effusion and a more complex septated effusion. Additionally, ultrasound can be used in the insertion of an intercostal catheter (ICC) for drainage of the effusion. Computed tomography is not routinely recommended for parapneumonic effusion, except in those cases where it may aid surgery or USS is unclear. Baseline bloods including blood cultures, white cell count, haemoglobin, platelets, and electrolytes are recommended. Daily chest X-ray and bloods to assess progress are not recommended. Diagnostic thoracentesis is not routinely performed in children but pleural fluid if drained should be sent off for culture and tested with enhanced molecular techniques such as PCR.

Treatment of empyema is based on the severity of the effusion and the presence of septations. It is recommended empyema be managed by a paediatric pulmonologist in conjunction with paediatric surgeons, usually at a tertiary centre with access to paediatric intensive care and paediatric surgical services.

Grade 1 and 2 effusions on ultrasound can often be managed medically, while grade 3–4 effusions should be referred to the paediatric surgeons for consideration of surgical management (Figure 11.2). Supportive therapy is the mainstay of treatment, in addition to antibiotics, with supplemental oxygen as required, fluid resuscitation and antipyretics/analgesia. Early mobilization and deep breathing/coughing are encouraged to assist in achieving a more rapid resolution. IV antibiotics should be used and directed towards the cultured organism. Until an organism is cultured, broad-spectrum coverage should be used including coverage for *S. aureus* and *S. pneumoniae* with consideration given for MRSA coverage if patient is from a community with high prevalence or identifies as ATSI. Consideration can be given to step down from IV antibiotics to oral after patient is afebrile for 24 hours. Duration of antibiotics should be for at least 7 days up to 6 weeks with no consensus on duration.

Pleural drainage should be used in patients with respiratory distress, a large effusion, and ongoing sepsis despite antibiotics treatment. In large effusions, drainage is essential for lung re-expansion. The use of ICC for drainage alone is not recommended as this usually results in the need for rescue surgical treatment.

The use of intercostal catheters with fibrinolytics (urokinase/alteplase) to cause breakdown the fibrin septations improving drainage of the effusion is an effective management strategy for the majority of cases. Studies have shown a reduced hospital length of stay when fibrinolytics are used compared to drainage alone, and a 90% successful treatment rate. Dosing is twice daily for 3 days or a total of six doses. The remaining 10% that failed fibrinolytic therapy require surgical intervention. Surgical intervention via video-assisted thoracoscopic surgery (VATS) is the recommended surgical technique for empyema, although more complex collections may be more effectively treated with mini-thoracotomy or thoracotomy.

Chest drains can be removed when drainage is less than 1–2 mL/kg over 24 hours. Chest X-ray should be performed after removal of the chest drain.

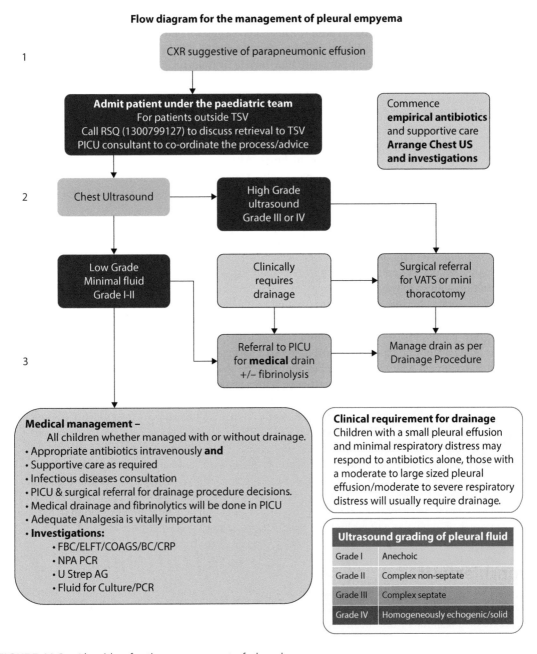

Flow diagram for the management of pleural empyema

1 CXR suggestive of parapneumonic effusion

Admit patient under the paediatric team
For patients outside TSV
Call RSQ (1300799127) to discuss retrieval to TSV
PICU consultant to co-ordinate the process/advice

Commence **empirical antibiotics** and supportive care **Arrange Chest US and investigations**

2 Chest Ultrasound

High Grade ultrasound Grade III or IV

Low Grade Minimal fluid Grade I–II

Clinically requires drainage

Surgical referral for VATS or mini thoracotomy

3 Referral to PICU for **medical** drain +/– fibrinolysis

Manage drain as per Drainage Procedure

Medical management –
All children whether managed with or without drainage.
• Appropriate antibiotics intravenously **and**
• Supportive care as required
• Infectious diseases consultation
• PICU & surgical referral for drainage procedure decisions.
• Medical drainage and fibrinolytics will be done in PICU
• Adequate Analgesia is vitally important
• **Investigations:**
  • FBC/ELFT/COAGS/BC/CRP
  • NPA PCR
  • U Strep AG
  • Fluid for Culture/PCR

Clinical requirement for drainage
Children with a small pleural effusion and minimal respiratory distress may respond to antibiotics alone, those with a moderate to large sized pleural effusion/moderate to severe respiratory distress will usually require drainage.

Ultrasound grading of pleural fluid	
Grade I	Anechoic
Grade II	Complex non-septate
Grade III	Complex septate
Grade IV	Homogeneously echogenic/solid

FIGURE 11.2 Algorithm for the management of pleural empyema.

Pulmonary Hydatid Disease

Hydatid disease is a zoonotic disease caused by the larvae of the family of parasite *Echinococcus*. The most common is *Echinococcus granulosus*, which causes cystic echinococcosis (CE) or cystic hydatid disease, which accounts for approximately 95% of cases globally. The most common site of infection worldwide is in the liver with pulmonary infection being the second most common. *E. granulosus* is endemic to Australia with many animals in Tropical North Australia playing host to the parasite. People who work with or are in regular close contact with animals are at increased risk for CE.

The lifecycle of *E. granulosus* has two stages. Adult worms live in the small intestine of definitive hosts such as carnivorous wild dogs. These worms release eggs which come out in definitive host faeces and are ingested by intermediate hosts (sheep, cattle, kangaroos, feral pigs). The eggs then hatch in the small intestine of the intermediate host where they invade the intestinal mucosa and spread systemically via blood or lymphatics, implanting into the organs and developing into hydatid cyst. The intermediate host ultimately respreads eggs back to the definitive host when they are eaten. Spread to human occurs via faecal-oral transmission from contaminated water, produce, or soil. In humans, the eggs evolve into parasitic embryos that attach to the wall of the duodenum or jejunum and penetrate the mucosa. They then reach the liver via the portal venous circulation and either attach here or continue via the inferior vena cava through the right heart settling in the lungs. Alternatively, embryos can reach the lungs via the thoracic duct to the internal jugular vein bypassing the hepatic system.

Once implanted, the embryos can start to form a hydatid cyst. Lung cysts grow faster than hepatic cysts due to the more elastic nature of pulmonary tissue.

Small cysts may remain asymptomatic and only be identified incidentally. Symptoms tend to occur when cysts grow large enough to cause mechanical effects on surrounding structures with cough being the most common symptom in children. Other sudden-onset symptoms may occur if a cyst ruptures such as: chest pain, hemoptysis, cough, a salty taste in mouth, and fevers. Cyst rupture may lead to a hypersensitivity reaction with anaphylaxis. When a pulmonary cyst is identified, liver ultrasound should always be performed to exclude hepatic involvement, isolated pulmonary cysts are more common in the paediatric population than in adults.

Cysts are commonly solitary and unilateral with the highest incidence in the right lower lobe. Diagnosis is via history of exposure to host animals, imaging, and serology.

Medical treatment with albendazole has shown to be an effective treatment for small cysts <5 cm in diameter. Larger cysts (>5 cm) are usually treated with a trial of albendazole with close monitoring to see if cyst size decreases; however, in a majority of cases, surgical resection of the cyst is required. The use of albendazole has the added benefit of creating a sterile cyst in case of secondary spillage intraoperatively. While using albendazole, liver function test should be checked fortnightly.

Multiple surgical techniques have been described for the treatment of pulmonary hydatid cysts. The standard approach is via a posterolateral thoracotomy with the aims of surgery being to remove the entire cyst while preserving lung parenchyma and avoiding intraoperative spillage. Cystostomy with capitonnage is the preferred method. Cystostomy involves aspiration of the cyst with complete removal of the germinal membrane and capitonnage reduces the risk of infection and empyema formation in the residual cavity. In cases of giant cyst and multiple cyst, lobectomy may be unavoidable.

Bronchiectasis

Bronchiectasis is a respiratory disease characterized by chronic infections leading to airway inflammation and progressive respiratory decline. Lower respiratory tract infections in the absence of underlying pathology account for the greatest number of cases of bronchiectasis. In most developed countries, bronchiectasis is rare. In the tropical areas of Northern Australia, with a higher population of Aboriginal and Torres Straight Islanders, bronchiectasis creates a significant burden on the health system. In this population without underlying conditions (specifically cystic fibrosis or alpha-1 antitrypsin deficiency), a severe lower respiratory tract infection early in life is believed to be the cause of bronchiectasis. The most common pathogens isolated in children are *H. influenzae*, *S. pneumoniae*, and *Moraxella catarrhalis*. In the ATSI populations of Tropical Australia, *S. aureus* is an important organism with increasing rates as the primary organism isolated.

The pathogenesis is an exaggerated inflammation in response to respiratory pathogens in a 'vicious circle' leading to tissue damage. In cases not responsive to treatment, the lungs may progress to having dilated airways increasing the work of breathing.

The primary treatment for bronchiectasis is with antibiotics. Antibiotic therapy is usually aimed at treating the most common causes of respiratory infections leading to bronchiectasis. At times, additional coverage with a macrolide, such as azithromycin, may be required to completely treat the infection. Additional treatment may consistent of the use of a mucolytic agent to assist in breaking up mucous in the lower airways to aid with clearance.

In rare cases of severe progression of disease, not responding to medical therapy, operative intervention may be required. Bronchoscopy may be used to relieve a blockage or clear mucus and take samples to better direct therapy. In rare cases, lobectomy may be required to remove the lobe effected by bronchiectasis. In cases of multilobar disease, treatment may progress all the way to a lung transplant.

BRONCHOPULMONARY MALFORMATIONS

Bronchopulmonary malformations (BPM) are a spectrum of developmental anomalies with a constantly evolving classification and nomenclature, believed to be from a common origin, but differ due to disparity in timing of development and/or position within the tracheobronchial tree.

Congenital Pulmonary Airway Malformation

Congenital pulmonary airway malformations (CPAMs), formerly known as congenital cystic adenomatoid malformations (CCAMs), are the most common form of BPM. Currently the incidence is estimated to be 1:2500 which is increased from previous estimates due to the advent of prenatal ultrasound picking up more lesions.

CPAMs are classified based on the Stocker classification looking at location, size, epithelial lining, and cystic structure (Table 11.4). More simply, they can be classified as microcystic or macrocystic based on size.

The blood supply to CPAMs comes from the pulmonary artery and pulmonary venous drainage. In rare cases, vascular supply can come from systemic vessels causing it to be confused for a bronchopulmonary sequestration (BPS) which is defined by having a systemic blood supply.

A vast majority of CPAMs are asymptomatic at birth, although large lesions can cause mass effect leading to mediastinal shift with compression of the lung or heart, interruption of the diaphragm with eversion, and in the most severe cases hydrops fetalis. Later in life, complications may arise as a result of infection of the malformation or rupture leading to pneumothorax.

Diagnosis is most commonly made prenatally with fetal ultrasound. Prenatally, if further differentiation is required (i.e. to exclude BPS or congenital diaphragmatic hernia), fetal MRI can be useful. When there is a prenatal diagnosis of CPAM, a chest radiograph should be performed shortly after birth. If the neonate is symptomatic or the chest radiograph shows large/bilateral/multifocal cyst/pneumothorax at

TABLE 11.4 Stocker classification of CPAMs

TYPE	CYST STRUCTURE	SIZE	EPITHELIAL LINING
0	Multiple	Differ	Ciliated pseudostratified columnar
1	Single/Multiple	>2 cm	Ciliated pseudostratified columnar
2	Multiple	<1 cm	Ciliated cuboidal/Columnar
3	Solid/Multiple scattered thin walled	<2 cm	Low cuboidal
4	Single/Multiple	Differs	Type 1 and 2 alveolar

birth, a CT or MRI should be completed. If the neonate is asymptomatic and does not show those features on a radiograph, a CT or MRI should still be performed although this is usually not urgent, which is usually preferable to be performed whilst a child can be wrapped and fed for a scan and avoiding a general anaesthetic where possible.

In cases of hydrops fetalis, CPAMs can be treated prenatally with fetal surgery, corticosteroids, or drainage, to prevent fetal termination. Postnatally, in symptomatic neonates, it is often possible to resect lesions thoracoscopically. Resections are additionally done in infants with lesions occupying >20% of the hemithorax, bilateral/multifocal cyst, pneumothorax, or a family history of pleuropulmonary blastoma. In older children, resection may be completed in order to prevent recurrent infections or if there is a malignancy risk (type 4 lesions). Controversy over what to do in asymptomatic CPAMs remains with resection or watch and wait both being reasonable options with the ultimate decision being made in conjunction with the family.

Bronchopulmonary Sequestration

BPS is non-functioning pulmonary tissue that derives its blood supply from the systemic circulation, with a majority of vascular supply coming from the aorta. BPS is either intra-lobar sequestration (ILS) or extra-lobar sequestration (ELS). ILS makes up approximately 75% of BPS and is found within the normal lung tissue lacking its own visceral pleura. ELS accounts for approximately 25% of BPS and is found outside the normal lung and has its own visceral pleura. ELS can be above, below, or in the diaphragm, with the majority being left sided and more commonly in males. The incidence of BPS is 0.15–6.4% of all congenital lung malformations.

Development is the result of supernumerary lobe bud development in foregut embryogenesis. The development of the bud in relation to the development of the pleura determines if it will be ILS or ELS. Development before the pleura leads to ILS, while development after the pleura results in EPS.

Diagnosis is primarily prenatal with ultrasonography. Doppler should be used to identify the arterial inflow to the lesion. A majority of those not picked up prenatally are picked up due to symptoms within the first 6 months of life, and a small percentage found incidentally later in life. Work-up is similar to that of CPAM, with the exception of CT angiography being the gold standard, in order to identify the systemic blood supply for surgical planning. Symptoms and management are also similar to that of CPAMs, with resection via thoracoscopy being indicated in symptomatic patients. Again resection in those who are asymptomatic is controversial; however, a vast majority advocate for resection.

Congenital Lobar Emphysema

Congenital lobar emphysema (CLE) is a condition of over expansion of one or more pulmonary lobes with histologically normal lung tissue and without destruction of alveolar walls. Air trapping during expiratory phase as a result of deficient bronchial cartilage leads to respiratory distress and making the lobe effectively non-functional. CLE has an estimated incidence of 1 in 20,000–30,000 live births occurring more commonly in males, with the largest number of cases effecting the left upper lobe (43%), followed by right middle lobe (32%), and right upper lobe (21%). An example of a left upper lobe CLE is seen in Figure 11.3.

Approximately 50% of patients are symptomatic at birth, with the majority of remaining cases being identified in the first 6 months of life. Common symptoms include difficulty with feeding/breathing, wheezing, and cyanosis. Breathing difficulties are a result of overinflated lungs leading to impaired ventilation and perfusion with progressive hyperinflation causing compression on adjacent structures.

- Evaluation with chest radiograph is the first step.
- CT is the gold standard for diagnosis of CLE.

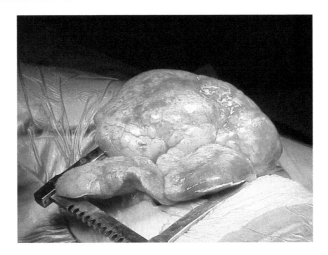

FIGURE 11.3   Left upper lobe congenital lobar emphysema.

Treatment is based on severity of symptoms. In mild and moderate cases, conservative management is the preferred choice. In patients with severe symptoms, the treatment of choice is lobectomy.

Bronchogenic Cysts

Bronchogenic cysts are foregut derivative cystic malformations that can be located ectopically anywhere along the foregut developmental pathway. They exhibit clinical and radiological polymorphism and can be confused for hydatid disease in endemic areas like Tropical Australia. They develop from abnormal/late budding of ventral lung bud or tracheobronchial tree. Location depends on stage of development with early development occupying the tracheobronchial tree and late development resulting in more peripheral lesions.

Classification of bronchogenic cysts is based upon their location.

Findings in children are usually secondary to infection or compression on surrounding structures which may cause life-threatening symptoms.

CT is the investigation of choice; however, MRI does provide better delineation of anatomic relationships and defining the cyst.

Surgery is indicated for symptomatic cyst via either thoracotomy or VATS. Intrapulmonary cysts should be resected via lobectomy.

Transport Considerations

It is important to remember that patients who have undergone thoracic surgery should not be transported by air unless absolutely necessary for a minimum of 3 weeks following surgery.

This includes normal domestic transfers which are quite commonplace in North Queensland because of the large distances involved travelling across the region. For patients being transferred with intrathoracic problems where there is the potential for air leak and tension pneumothorax, careful preparation and due consideration of the risk to be taken during transfer are necessary. In particular, it may become necessary to insert an intercostal drain or intubate a patient during transfer and appropriately trained staff and equipment should be available for transfer.

Miscellaneous Conditions

Chylothorax

Chylothorax is the accumulation of lymphatic fluid within the thoracic pleura. Chylothorax is broken into non-traumatic (congenital, neoplastic, infectious), traumatic (postoperative, blunt/penetrating injuries), and idiopathic with traumatic making up more than 50% of all cases based on more recent data. In the paediatric population, the prevalence is estimated to be 1 per 15,000 deliveries and a risk of 0.2–2% post-operatively in paediatric thoracic operations.

Symptoms are usually the result of mechanical compression on pulmonary expansion resulting in breathlessness. Evaluation with chest radiograph is routinely done but cannot differentiate chylothorax from a pleural effusion. MRI is the only imaging modality that can confidently confirm cisterna chyli. Thoracentesis and analysis of the fluid is diagnostic with high level of lymphocytes and triglycerides >110 mg/dL.

In the majority of cases, treatment is conservative/medical for chylothorax/chyle like disease with dietary changes and use of somatostatin. Surgical intervention is reserved for cases that fail medical management and instances where intercostal catheter output is greater than 50 mL/kg/day.

Foreign Bodies

Ingested foreign bodies are a common emergency room presentation with 80% of presentations being in the paediatric population. Coins are the most frequently swallowed oesophageal foreign body in children, followed by food objects (fish bones, chicken wings). It is most common in children for ingested foreign bodies to become stuck at the lower end of the oesophagus. Only around 40% of objects will be completely asymptomatic; however, most foreign bodies will pass through the gastrointestinal system without intervention. Ten to twenty per cent will require medical intervention (oesophagoscopy) and 1% or less will require surgical management.

Foreign bodies that require urgent management include those causing oesophageal obstruction (unable to tolerate secretions), button batteries, and sharp-pointed objects in the oesophagus.

Evaluation with chest radiograph is recommended to confirm the presence of foreign body in the oesophagus. AP and lateral views may be required in order to assess for the 'double halo' sign of a button battery.

Button batteries cause damage by a mucosa bridge of positive and negative terminals leading to completion of the circuit allowing for flow of the charge. This in term leads to the formation of hydroxide radicals causing caustic injury with associated coagulation necrosis. **Current recommendations are to provide 10 ml of honey every 10 minutes up to 6 doses**, to help neutralize the discharging current, until the button battery can be removed. This comes with the risk of botulism if too much honey is provided and is not recommended in children under 12 months of age.

The most feared complication of button battery ingestion is an aorto-oesophageal fistula, with the greatest risk being in children younger than 5 years of age. The risk is increased in this age group due to more delayed presentation post ingestion. Additional significant complications include oesophageal perforation, stricture, vertebral osteomyelitis, and spondylodiscitis.

SUMMARY

Thoracic surgery is uncommon in childhood but in tropical areas a number of conditions are more commonly seen. In particular, the progression of pneumonia to a complex pneumonia complicated by lung abscesses and the development of parapneumonic effusions is much more common. This is likely related not only to the delays in treatment and lack of access to healthcare services for remotely located patients as well as medical treatment failures due to a difference in the microbiological ecosystem seen in tropical areas. It is important to initiate early aggressive medical management of patients with LRTI who are failing to respond to medical management. Patients may need to be transferred to hospitals with PICU/respiratory paediatric support and surgical expertise for successful management and this is preferably prior to deterioration as aero-retrieval can be more difficult in patients who have respiratory compromise is not straightforward. A more complete understanding of the role of more aggressive therapies such as fibrinolytic usage will hopefully be forthcoming as experience of their usage grows.

FURTHER READING

Dehner LP, Hill DA, Deschryver K. Pathology of the breast in children, adolescents, and young adults. Semin Diagn Pathol. 1999 August;16(3):235–47.

Gautam A, Wiseman GG, Goodman ML, Ahmedpour S, Lindsay D, Heyer A, Stalewski H, Norton RE, White AV. Paediatric thoracic empyema in the tropical North Queensland region of Australia: Epidemiological trends over a decade. J Paediatr Child Health. 2018 July;54(7):735–40.

Gautam A, Wiseman G, Legg R, Lindsay D, Puvvadi R, Rathnamma BM, Stalewski H, Norton R, White AV. Management of pediatric thoracic empyema in the North Queensland region of Australia and impact of a local evidence-based treatment guideline. Pediatr Infect Dis J. 2022 January;41(1):1–5.

Leung AKC, Leung AAC. Gynecomastia in infants, children, and adolescents. Recent Pat Endocr Metab Immune Drug Discov. 2017;10(2):127–37.

Limaiem F, Mlika M. Bronchogenic cyst. 2022 Jul:5. In: StatPearls [Internet]. Treasure Island (FL): StatPearls Publishing; 2022 January.

Nabi MS, Waseem T. Pulmonary hydatid disease: What is the optimal surgical strategy? Int J Surg. 2010;8(8):612–6.

Obermeyer RJ, Goretsky MJ. Chest wall deformities in pediatric surgery. Surg Clin North Am. 2012 June;92(3): 669–84, ix.

Sethia R, Gibbs H, Jacobs IN, Reilly JS, Rhoades K, Jatana KR. Current management of button battery injuries. Laryngoscope Investing Otolaryngol. 2021 April;6(3):549–63.

Wong KKY, Flake AW, Tibboel D, Rottier RJ, Tam PKH. Congenital pulmonary airway malformation: Advances and controversies. Lancet Child Adolesc Health. 2018 April;2(4):290–7.

Emergency Abdominal Surgery in Children

12

Daniel Carroll

INTRODUCTION

The mainstay of paediatric surgical practice is abdominal surgery. A number of important conditions have already been discussed elsewhere within this book, but this chapter aims to examine in more detail the surgery for the common pathologies seen in our practice.

SURGERY FOR APPENDICITIS

Appendicitis is common. It is not unusual for patients to present to our regional centre after the diagnosis of appendicitis has already been made. It is important to correlate the findings of investigations with the clinical picture to try and ensure the correct diagnosis is made prior to taking the patient to theatre. Unfortunately, some tests which are commonly requested such as ultrasound scan (USS) have a poor sensitivity and specificity in children if performed in centres with limited experience in paediatric ultrasonography and if used indiscriminately it does not help in coming to a correct diagnosis. We have already discussed the management of appendicitis in Chapter 7. The principles of management are resuscitation and stabilisation of the patient, expeditious transfer and then surgery. In patients with suspected appendicitis, surgery can be performed by a non-specialist paediatric surgeon. In our practice, we are fortunate that our colleagues in other regional centres will often manage patients with appendicitis without the need for involvement of paediatric surgical services. This is particularly useful in keeping patients close to home where family support is often available as well as reducing the demand on transport services. Where patients cannot be managed locally then they are transferred to our service, this may be for a variety of reasons; the child may have other complex medical needs; they may be too young to be operated on locally; they may require paediatric intensive care if very unwell; there may be no surgeon/anaesthetist available locally.

An Approach to Operative Management

Once the diagnosis is confirmed, then the patient is commenced on appropriate fluids and intravenous antibiotics should be commenced. This should be at least 1 h prior to theatre wherever possible. It is important to examine the child carefully to look for the presence of an abdominal mass. Patients with an appendix mass may be treated conservatively in the first instance. The operation for appendix masses may be difficult and

DOI: 10.1201/9781003156659-12

better results are often achieved by treatment with intravenous antibiotics and improving the clinical condition of the patient with a delayed interval appendicectomy. This is the best course of action in patients with a contained mass where there is not widespread peritonitis and the patient is improving and able to tolerate diet. Patients who do not improve with antibiotics, who become peritonitic, or who cannot tolerate feeds may need an operation but it should be approached with circumspection and wherever possible a senior surgeon should be present or aware of the case as the potential for conversion to an open procedure is there. It is usual in such cases for preparations to made for intensive care support postoperatively, blood should be ordered, and theatre teams and the anaesthetic team should know about the potential for conversion to laparotomy.

The majority of patients with appendicitis present in a more straightforward manner. Appendicitis is commonest in children between the age of 10 and 16 years. These patients often present with the classical signs of localising abdominal tenderness and guarding. Simple observations usually show a low-grade temperature and where there are doubts about the diagnosis a white cell count will usually be elevated in patients with appendicitis although the specificity of this as a stand-alone test is low. Other conditions such as mesenteric adenitis and urinary tract infections will commonly mimic appendicitis, particularly in younger children. There are two major operative approaches, but most surgeons elect to perform a laparoscopic appendicectomy in the first instance.

Laparoscopic Appendicectomy

Most patients are best treated with a laparoscopic appendicectomy. The equipment required even in small children is now readily available, often children are as large as adult patients but generally we use 5 mm ports for both the camera and the instruments. Smaller 3 mm ports are available for smaller patients.

The first step is the treatment after establishing the diagnosis and managing the fluids and antibiotics. Once a child is stable, then surgery is indicated. Whilst we no longer operate emergently on children, we try to perform surgery as soon as practical. It is not usual to operate between midnight and first light unless the child is very unwell as often patients benefit from more conservative management prior to theatre and the availability of other staff in the event of unexpected problems can be problematic. Multiple studies into the management of surgical problems have demonstrated better outcomes for patients in avoiding emergent operations. Consent should be taken from the parents. It is important to discuss the potential complications with families prior to surgery.

Consent for Laparoscopic Appendicectomy

It is important to be able to explain clearly to the family the reasons for the surgery, the expected outcomes and the risks of common complications. Only after the family understands the risks and benefits of the procedure can meaningful informed consent be obtained. It is important to check that families understand the procedure, and this step is often overlooked or performed poorly.

Potential Risks

- Normal appendix (5–10%)
- Surgical site infection (1–5%)
- Intra-abdominal collection
- Bleeding requiring re-operation or transfusion
- Conversion to open appendicectomy
- Need for additional tests or further procedures
- Scars
- Faecal fistula
- Adhesions

LAPAROSCOPIC APPENDICECTOMY – OPERATIVE STEPS

The *aim* of the procedure is to safely remove the appendix, identify and exclude any other pathologies and to washout any infection in the peritoneal cavity.

After performing the necessary WHO checks and confirming the consent and checking the equipment, the patient is positioned in a supine position with both arms tucked at the sides (in larger children, it may be necessary to put the arms on boards). If the bladder is full or if advanced appendicitis is expected, then a Foley catheter and a naso-gastric tube (NGT) are inserted.

The patient's entire abdomen is then prepped and draped. Once the laparoscopic equipment has been checked and permission to proceed has been gained from the anaesthetist, it is necessary to visualise the appendix. We perform this by initially placing a camera through a small incision just underneath the umbilicus. It is usual for us to do this as an open (Hassan) procedure in children rather than using a Veress needle. The abdomen is much more elastic in small children and it is possible to cause vascular injuries in children from using a Veress needle. Careful opening of the umbilicus and entry into the peritoneal cavity are necessary to reduce the risk of injury to underlying structures.

Once the camera port is inserted, then insufflation is performed with carbon dioxide. It is colourless, inexpensive and non-flammable. In addition, it has higher blood solubility than air which reduces the risk of complications if venous embolism occurs. A usual starting flow rate of 2 L/min and a pressure of 10 mmHg are usually a safe starting point for the settings although it may be necessary to increase the flow rate and pressure in larger children. Once the abdomen begins to expand, then the camera is focussed and white balanced. The scope can be warmed to prevent condensation, or an antifogging agent is used. It is most usual to use a 30-degree angled scope for the procedure and a skilled camera assistant makes the procedure much easier.

Once the camera is introduced, we inspect the right lower quadrant and, if possible, confirm the appendix is indeed the cause of the pain. Once this has been done, then two 5 mm ports are introduced. If the bladder is full, it may be necessary to empty the bladder by expression or passing a urethral catheter which has not been done already. One port is introduced to the left lower quadrant. I like to infiltrate with local anaesthetic and pierce the peritoneum with the needle prior to inserting a blunt port after blunt dissection using scissors. As stated previously, the peritoneum is much more elastic in small children and it is possible to create serious injuries using sharp ports. Careful insertion of ports is an important operative skill for surgeons to master.

Once the first operating port is inserted, it is possible to use instruments to stabilise the anterior abdominal wall from the inside during insertion of the second port which often makes this easier. The second port should be placed just above and lateral to the bladder. The bladder is relatively a much larger structure in small children and recognising this prior to attempting the ports is an important safety measure. Once two ports are inserted, the appendix can be grasped and removed. Usually, it is retrieved using a bag and if the appendix is inflamed then the peritoneal cavity should be irrigated with copious volumes of warmed saline.

Operative Pitfalls

It is important to acknowledge the differences in anatomy between small children and young adults. Small children have a much larger distance laterally across the abdomen than they do in the midline. The liver can come down much lower than expected and the bladder sits higher. It is important to examine the child once anaesthetised as it is possible to feel a large mass that may have not been clear prior to anaesthesia. On such occasions, it is necessary to consider whether progression with surgery is appropriate and discussion with a senior surgeon is useful. An appendix abscess is often best treated with parenteral antibiotics and an interval appendicectomy. Other masses may represent more serious underlying pathology such as malignancy and it is wise to be prepared for the potential need to convert an open operation.

On rare occasions, other pathology may be demonstrated. A number of conditions mimic appendicitis. Enlarged, inflamed lymph nodes from mesenteric adenitis cause pain when pushed into contact with peritoneum. A large number of important lymph nodes are located around the mesentery of the terminal ileum and their position close to the appendix is the commonest cause of diagnostic confusion. Large lymph nodes may represent more sinister pathology. Lymph nodes that are greater than 1 cm in diameter may be pathological but clinical correlation is required, including careful examination for other nodes and evaluation of B symptoms (fever, night sweats and weight loss). Children can often have marked lymphadenopathy in response to viral illnesses. It is possible for enlarged lymphatic tissues (either mesenteric lymph nodes or enlarged Peyer's patches) to act as a pathological lead point resulting in an intussusception. Patients with intussusception found at laparoscopy for suspected appendicitis should undergo laparoscopic reduction where possible and then further assessment for a pathological lead-point. It may be necessary to convert to an open procedure to reduce the intussuscipiens and resect bowel if it is not viable. The threshold for conversion to an open procedure is often dependent upon the experience of the surgeon with laparoscopic procedures.

If the appendix is normal, it is important to check for other pathologies. In girls and young women, ovarian pathologies can mimic appendicitis and the pelvis should be inspected and the presence of normal ovaries and fallopian tubes should be confirmed and recorded in the operation note. In all children, it is possible for a Meckel's diverticulum to become inflamed. Meckel's diverticulitis can result in perforation or painless bleeding. It is often possible to perform a laparoscopic-assisted procedure where the small bowel is delivered via the umbilicus and the Meckel's diverticulum is removed. If there is any bleeding from ectopic gastric mucosa, it is important to remember that this occurs away from the Meckel's diverticulum usually downstream from the diverticulum. For symptomatic Meckel's diverticulum, it is often necessary to resect a small portion of small bowel and perform an end-to-end anastomosis.

In a very small number of children, it is possible to identify inflammatory bowel disease at the time of laparoscopic appendicectomy. The appendix should be taken for histopathology which will often help make a diagnosis of Crohn's disease. These patients require careful watching after surgery as the risk of fistula and adhesions is much higher. Fortunately, it is uncommon for children to present in this way.

Intra-abdominal malignancy may also present as peritonitis. Often there are other symptoms which point to this diagnosis, particularly a long period of illness and weight loss. Rarely a wide variety of solid tumours can present with peritonitis, classically a ruptured Wilms' tumour presents in an acutely unwell child with peritonitis.

Removal of Ports

Once the operation is complete, I like to remove ports under direct vision to ensure that no omentum becomes entrapped in the port site. The final port to remove is the camera port. Small 3–5 mm port sites do not need to be closed other than at the skin level. I like to formally close the infraumbilical camera port with 3/0 vicryl to the deeper layers and with 4/0 caprosyn to the skin incisions.

Postoperative Management

For uncomplicated appendicitis, it is possible for patients to commence on fluids and diet as tolerated soon after the procedure. They should be encouraged to mobilise as soon as practical and appropriate and adequate pain relief is essential in helping to achieve this goal. Shoulder tip pain from retained carbon dioxide irritating the diaphragm is common and mobilisation helps the gas to reabsorb more quickly. For patients with necrotic or gangrenous appendicitis, it is necessary to continue parenteral antibiotics for longer. I like to ensure patients have been apyrexial for a minimum of 48 h and are improving clinically before stopping antibiotics. Those patients with complicated appendicitis should receive triple antibiotics (a penicillin, gentamicin and metronidazole). Local antibiotic policies should be adhered as should the principle of good antimicrobial stewardship. It is important to check operative specimens for antibiotic resistance. Children often require encouragement to eat following surgery, and the involvement of the dietician to ensure adequate calories are being taken can be useful. A nasogastric tube is often very useful in patients with a prolonged ileus after complicated appendicitis as it allows the surgeon to judge an appropriate time to recommence feeds. Generally younger patients are not at risk of deep-vein thrombosis (DVT) and require no specific safeguards to prevent this, but in larger patients (particularly post-pubertal girls), it may be necessary to consider DVT prophylaxis in a similar manner to adult patients.

Follow-Up Arrangements and Discharge Instructions

It is important to check the pathology for unexpected findings. Very rarely tumours of the appendix (e.g. carcinoid) may be seen. These patients require further investigations and additional management involving the paediatric oncology service. More commonly, we find evidence of worms which require treatment for the patient and for the entire family unit. Patients are discharged once they have clinically improved and are able to be cared for at home by the family. In uncomplicated appendicitis, this can be within 24 h. Those patients who live more remotely may benefit from a slightly extended stay outside of hospital in local accommodation prior to returning to a remote setting. It is important to keep the dressings dry and clean and look for signs of surgical site infection as well giving parents appropriate advice to reattend if the child becomes unwell, fails to recover or worsens at home. Contact sport and swimming should be avoided for 2 weeks. The patients can be followed up using telehealth for remote and regional patients around 4–6 weeks after surgery.

Damage Control Laparotomy

Whilst the principles of damage control surgery are the same in children as in adults, some important differences should be considered. Fortunately, the need for damage control surgery is very rare. Often patients with significant intra-abdominal injuries have other systems involved, and it is unusual to present with isolated injuries. The management of trauma in children is considered in Chapter 8. Unfortunately, we do see isolated intra-abdominal injuries in the context of inflicted or non-accidental injuries in children. In such cases, the injuries can be extensive. Wherever possible, it is almost always useful to gain an idea of the extent and location of the injuries prior to surgery and a CT scan is almost always useful and can be performed as resuscitation continues if necessary. On a handful of occasions, we will need to operate without access to any imaging, and in such cases, a structured and methodical approach to surgery is useful.

Preoperative Preparation

Wherever possible, it is important to involve paediatric anaesthesia, other surgical teams and paediatric intensive care colleagues to provide support and advice as needed both preoperatively and intraoperatively. For a damage control laparotomy, it is usual to allow the PICU/Paediatric Anaesthetic team to prepare for a massive transfusion protocol.

Damage Control Surgery

Damage control surgery consists of three steps:

- Abbreviated surgery to control the haemorrhage and contamination
- Resuscitation in the ICU
- Planned re-operation and definitive surgery

A better understanding of the pathophysiology of the coagulopathic response in trauma has led to the move to address coagulopathy during resuscitation. In balanced resuscitation, fluid administration is restricted and hypotension is allowed until haemostatic measures begin. The administration of blood products is recommended early in resuscitation.

Massive Transfusion Protocol

Massive transfusion is typically defined as the transfusion of 10 or more units of packed red blood cells within the first 24 h of injury.

The beneficial effects of the implementation of the MTP have been reported by several authors. It requires a team-based approach and is best when initiated early in resuscitation.

Initial Approach to Surgery

Once the patient has been stabilised as much as possible and a joint decision has been made to proceed to emergency surgery, the patient is consented and taken to theatre expeditiously. Most hospitals have a 'red blanket' code allowing for immediate entry into theatre with appropriately trained staff and availability of equipment.

Patient Positioning and Preparation and Incision

The patient is positioned supine and the abdomen generously prepped to allow extension of the incision into the chest if necessary. Once all the equipment and the anaesthetist are ready, it is most normal to perform a midline incision from the xiphisternum to the pubis. As the abdomen is opened, it is important to be ready to try and recycle any blood loss using a cell saver where available which must be set up prior to making the incision. As the abdomen is opened, it may result in catastrophic blood loss and cardiac arrest.

Abbreviated Surgery

Once the abdomen is open, it is necessary to pack all four quadrants with large packs to stop active bleeding. It may be necessary to utilise more than one assistant at this stage. Once the bleeding is controlled by direct pressure, then the blood is evacuated and a careful inspection of all four quadrants is performed. It is usual to start in quadrants where there is least likely to be major bleeding and then to pack these areas off again before moving to areas where more involved surgery may be necessary.

Sometimes it is not possible to progress beyond packing of the abdomen and in such instances, it may be necessary to return the patient to PICU for further resuscitation with an open abdomen. This can be controlled with a number of packs and then a large occlusive dressing. If suction is then placed underneath the drain and a reasonable seal is achieved, this can further splint the abdomen as a temporising measure.

In the event of major liver or vascular injuries, the specialist adult surgeons usually assist in the surgery. Injuries of the mesentery, the kidneys or the spleen can usually be dealt with by a general paediatric surgeon.

INTUSSUSCEPTION

Intussusception has already been discussed in Chapter 6; however, a description of the necessary steps in operation and potential pitfalls are outlined in the following sections.

Introduction

Intussusception is usually managed by pneumatic or hydrostatic reduction. In cases where this is contraindicated (e.g. perforation) or where this fails, it may be necessary to perform open or laparoscopic surgery.

Consent for Laparotomy for Intussusception

It is important to consider and carefully explain the reason for surgery to the family. On some occasions, the child is either too unwell to attempt radiological reduction and in some older children such attempts are not possible. In our patients, it is often the case that transfer difficulties mean that patients present after much longer time periods than those usually seen in metropolitan practice.

A failed radiological reduction does not automatically result in surgery, as a partial reduction of an ileo-colic intussusception in a well child allows for a period of rest and continued conservative management and a further attempt a few hours later. Likewise, a recurrent intussusception does not necessitate an operation but may point to a pathological lead point that will require surgery. The major indications for surgery are as follows:

- Peritonitis
- Perforation
- Failed reduction
- Unstable child
- Pathological lead point

The surgeon should discuss with families the reason for progressing to surgery, including the risks of open and laparoscopic surgery. Different surgeons have preferences for open or laparoscopic surgery, and they will often commence the surgery laparoscopically and progress to an open or laparoscopic-assisted procedure. It is important to discuss the risk of complications, including the potential need for stoma formation, the possibility of bowel resection and the potential finding of a pathological lead-point due to malignancy, e.g. lymphoma. The short-term complications include infection and bleeding, and the long-term complications include adhesions and the need for further surgeries.

Surgery for Intussusception

Once resuscitation has been commenced including placement of an NGT and administration of intravenous fluids and antibiotics has commenced, then the patient should be taken to theatre. After a routine WHO check, the patient is positioned supine and the abdomen prepped to allow access to the whole abdomen. If the child is unwell or a laparoscopic approach is intended, it is usual to place a Foley's catheter at this stage to monitor urine output and reduce the risk of bladder injury during laparoscopy. For an open approach, it is normal to make a transverse infra-umbilical right-sided incision to allow access to the ileo-caecal region.

If there is an intussusception, it should be carefully and gently reduced and then the bowel inspected for viability. It may be necessary to warm the bowel for several minutes to re-establish a good blood supply. Once this has been done, it is necessary to look for a lead point and determine if there is a pathological lead point that needs to be removed. If so, it is usual to have to remove bowel with the pathological lead point and perform an end-to-end small bowel anastomosis. It is often possible to reduce the intussusception laparoscopically by gentle traction on the bowel, and surprisingly it is not uncommon for the intussusception to spontaneously reduce with the administration of anaesthesia.

If there are large (pathological) lymph nodes, it may be necessary to perform a lymph node biopsy to exclude lymphoma.

Pitfalls in practice

It is vitally important to ensure the patient is adequately resuscitated prior to commencing surgery. Once the intussusception is reduced, the return of blood flow to the bowel can result in profound and sudden hypotension. It is important that the family are prepared for a potential admission to PICU postoperatively and that the PICU team are aware of the patient prior to surgery.

Wherever possible, it is ideal to gain as much information as possible about the presence of a pathological lead-point prior to surgery to guide conversations with the family.

SUMMARY

There are many potential reasons for emergency paediatric surgical intervention; however, outside of neonatal surgery, it is fortunately unusual to have to perform emergency surgery. The three most common surgeries are for appendicitis (common but usually straightforward), trauma (fortunately rare) and intussusception. Despite their differences, one common theme running through the management of all these conditions is the need to come to a timely diagnosis and formulate a management strategy and to adequately resuscitate a patient prior to theatre and wherever to anticipate problems before they arise.

The major mistakes in management arise from inadequate preparation for theatre and insufficient planning for major complications. The move away from emergent surgery by junior doctors without supervision has greatly reduced the incidence of these complications.

FURTHER READING

Bogert JN, Harvin JA, Cotton BA. Damage control resuscitation. J Intensive Care Med. 2016 March;31(3):177–86.

Glass CC, Rangel SJ. Overview and diagnosis of acute appendicitis in children. Semin Pediatr Surg. 2016 August;25(4):198–203.

Gluckman S, Karpelowsky J, Webster AC, McGee RG. Management for intussusception in children. Cochrane Database Syst Rev. 2017 June;6(6):CD006476.

Hamill J. Damage control surgery in children. Injury. 2004 July;35(7):708–12.

Stringer MD. Acute appendicitis. J Paediatr Child Health. 2017 November;53(11):1071–6.

Problems with the External Genitalia

13

Helen Buschel and Daniel Carroll

INTRODUCTION

The appearance and problems with the external genitalia of children are common causes for parents to seek medical attention. In our practice, almost one in four paediatric surgical appointments are given for concerns about the position of the testes or of problems with the foreskin. An understanding of the normal appearance of the external genitalia in male and female infants is essential in any medical practice. Recognising pathology is important in allowing for appropriate and expeditious treatment of problems that do occur. It is often helpful to consider abnormalities of the external genitalia as either congenital or acquired. In practice, however, the most significant pathology should be identified in the neonatal period. It is convenient to divide problems into those concerning boys and girls separately and to further consider problems as either congenital or acquired.

CONGENITAL PROBLEMS

Assessment of the External Genitalia of the Infant

An essential component of the neonatal check is to ensure that the genitals are normal, and that the testes are palpable and adequately descended. When they are noted to be abnormal, it is often a cause of serious concern and considerable anxiety for families. Congenital abnormalities of the normal development of the penis are present in around 1 in 200 live births and abnormalities of testicular descent are detected in around 1 in 60 male infants at 1 year of age. Overall, around 2% of male infants have abnormalities of the external genitalia.

Sexual Differentiation

Sexual differentiation is dependent upon the expression of the SRY gene, located on the Y chromosome; the gene products of the SRY gene stimulate the medullary sex cords to differentiate into secretory pre-Sertoli cells. From around the 7th week of gestation, these cells produce anti-Mullerian hormone (AMH) which plays a central role in the development of the male phenotype. The paramesonephric ducts

DOI: 10.1201/9781003156659-13

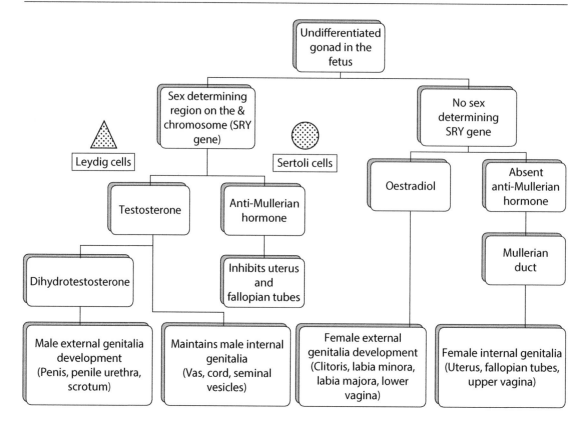

FIGURE 13.1   Simplified schematic of sexual differentiation.

disappear leaving behind only the appendix testis and utriculus. At the same time, Leydig cells in the primitive testes produce testosterone. This is converted by the action of 5-alpha reductase to form dihydrotestosterone which drives the growth and normal development of the male external genitalia. In the male foetus, the urogenital sinus advances onto the developing phallus as the urethral groove; subsequently this canalises to form the anterior urethra and closure of the urethra should be completed by 15 weeks of gestation. In the absence of adequate expression of the SRY gene or effective androgen production or sensitivity, the external genitalia progress down the pathway of female development. The genital tubercle becomes the clitoris, the urogenital sinus becomes the labia minora and the labioscrotal folds persist as the labia majora. These processes are summarised in Figure 13.1.

PROBLEMS WITH THE MALE GENITALIA

Abnormalities of Testicular Descent

The most common congenital abnormality of the external genitalia is cryptorchidism. In the male neonate, the testis should be present bilaterally and it is usually easy to draw the testis to the base of a well-developed scrotum. In infants, the testis is usually 1–2 mL in volume and roughly the same volume as the glans penis. Testicular descent occurs in two distinct phases. The first phase (abdominal phase) is initiated by the presence of AMH and its actions on the gubernaculum, which extends down to the labioscrotal folds; a second more active phase of testicular descent begins towards the end of the second trimester.

Under the influence of testosterone, the gubernaculum contracts, drawing the testis into its definitive scrotal position. Abnormal positioning of the gubernaculum leads to an ectopically positioned testis, impaired testosterone production or testosterone recognition results in testicular maldescent. Further spontaneous testicular descent is unusual after 3 months of age, as circulating levels of androgens fall dramatically and do not start to rise again until the onset of puberty.

Up to 1:30 boys undergo operations for inadequately descended testes in some series, although the incidence of testicular maldescent in the first year of life when assessed by specialist paediatric surgeons is only 1:60. Some boys have an adequate scrotal testicular position as an infant but as the child grows the testis remains stationary in relation to the external ring and thus occupy a less satisfactory scrotal position as time goes on (this is sometimes termed the ascending testis – although the author believes a more appropriate term should be the stationary testis). It is clear from the complicated nature of the processes driving normal testicular descent (which have been simplified here) that there are a wide variety of different causes of testicular maldescent; a deep understanding of the pathology is fortunately not required in everyday practice.

Classification of Abnormalities of Testicular Descent

Abnormally descended testes can be described as either palpable (80%) or impalpable (20%). Palpable undescended testes are more common and are described according to the position of the testis in relation to the base of the scrotum. The majority are found in the superficial inguinal pouch and can often be swept into the scrotum during clinical examination in a contented infant. Occasionally testes occupy an ectopic position. Patients presenting with impalpable testes present more of a challenge. In some cases, the testes are absent, some are completely intra-abdominal and a smaller number are within the inguinal canal. Boys with impalpable gonads may have more complex disorders of sexual differentiation. The combination of abnormalities of the penis and impalpable testes warrants prompt further investigations and urgent referral to a specialist centre. In practice, it is important to differentiate between impalpable and undescended or ectopic testes. Those boys with impalpable testes require further assessment and investigation and usually require more involved and staged surgical treatment. Differentiating between retractile and truly undescended testes can also be difficult and often confused by inappropriate use of investigations such as ultrasound scanning. A *retractile testis* can often be found sitting in the superficial inguinal pouch and can be drawn into the scrotum without tension and stays there upon release. These boys typically have descended testes noted at birth and then present to the GP with concerns about the testes being absent at a later age. Parents will often report that the testes can be seen when in a warm bath and the scrotum is typically normally developed. In these boys, the presence of the normal cremasteric reflex draws the testes out of the scrotum when the boy is cold, frightened or crying and this often happens when the clothes or nappy are removed in small children. Whilst boys with truly retractile testes usually do not require surgery, it is important to consider that around 1:10 of these boys ultimately go on to have an unsatisfactory scrotal position of the testis in childhood and so should be followed up carefully as they grow.

Normal Anatomy and Development of the Penis

The male external genitalia are a complex structure. The penis is composed of three tubes; dorsally the two corpora cavernosa sit above a third tube, the corpus spongiosum, which contains the urethra. Hypospadias is not a single distinct entity but rather a range of abnormalities involving the abnormal development of the corpora spongiosum. In the most severe forms of hypospadias, the corpora spongiosum is absent resulting in a perineal urethral opening. The more profound variants of hypospadias are fortunately rare, but consideration of disorders of sexual differentiation must be given when they are seen at birth, as this can be a medical emergency. These boys require urgent assessment, and particular note should be made of the presence or absence of adequately descending testicles. Profound hypospadias is also associated with a number of syndromes, so a complete and thorough clinical examination and detailed history taking are vital prior to deciding whether any further investigations are required. This can be a worrying time for families and prompt evaluation and referral to specialist centres is important.

HYPOSPADIAS

In the majority of cases, the external signs of hypospadias are obvious at birth but can be missed if a hasty or incomplete examination of the external genitalia is made. It is important for children with hypospadias to be detected early as this allows for a detailed explanation of the condition to be made to the parents and appropriate surgical management to be initiated before the child is 2 years of age. This is important as it means the child can undergo reconstructive surgery prior to being continent.

Clinical Features of Hypospadias

There are five distinct components to hypospadias, and these are all important in the assessment of the condition as well as indicating the likely underlying aetiology of the condition.

The cardinal feature of hypospadias is an ectopic urethral opening which can occur anywhere from the perineum through to glans. The normal or orthotopic urethral meatus is slit-like in appearance and located at the tip of the penis. Minor abnormalities of the position of the urethral meatus are quite common, but if the foreskin is intact at birth, these are often not appreciated until children are older. Fortunately, minor positional abnormalities of the urethral opening are not usually a cause for concern and parents should be reassured that functionally and aesthetically there is no need for surgical correction. Sometimes hypospadias is noted at the time of an elective circumcision for either religious or cultural reasons. In this instance, it is important that the child is not circumcised until a thorough assessment of the hypospadias is made by a paediatric urologist, as circumcision is contraindicated.

Classification of Hypospadias

Commonly hypospadias is classified according to the position of the meatus in relation to the ventral surface. Perhaps most useful for the non-surgeon, it can be divided into *distal* (85%) or *proximal* (15%) hypospadias.

The most distal form of hypospadias is *glanular*. Here the urethral meatus opens onto the glans itself. The most common form of hypospadias is where the opening is positioned at the junction of the glans and the shaft of the penis. This is *subcoronal* hypospadias (see Figure 13.2). These two forms of distal hypospadias comprise 80–85% of all cases of hypospadias. They are not usually associated with other problems and remain the most straightforward forms of hypospadias to correct surgically.

As the opening becomes more proximal, it can be described as *distal-shaft* or *mid-shaft* hypospadias. Although these forms of hypospadias are less common, they are still often amenable to a single-stage operation to correct the abnormality. Care must be taken in assessing these infants, as the hypospadias can be more severe than it appears at casual inspection and assessing for other genital abnormalities is important.

Proximal hypospadias describes an opening close to the junction of the penile shaft and the scrotum, and where it occurs proximal to this, it may be described as *penoscrotal or scrotal*. The most severe form of hypospadias is where the opening sits outside the scrotum within the perineum. This *perineal* hypospadias is often associated with scrotal abnormalities, most commonly a bifid scrotum. Fortunately, such extreme forms of hypospadias are rare and require specialist reconstruction and assessment. The different forms of hypospadias are shown in Figure 13.3.

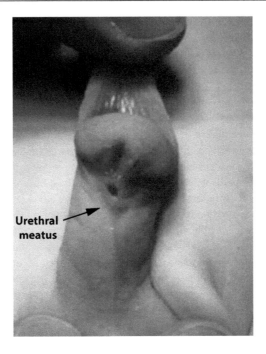

FIGURE 13.2   Subcoronal hypospadias.

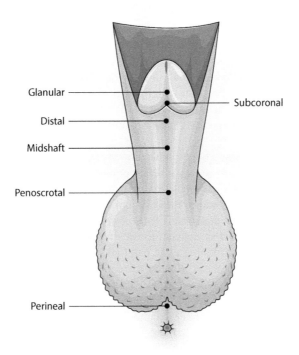

FIGURE 13.3   Classification of hypospadias.

The second feature of hypospadias is not universal; however, in its absence, it is not possible to detect the hypospadias at birth. The foreskin is usually incomplete on the ventral surface, giving rise to what is described as a *hooded foreskin*. Hypospadias in the absence of this defect is termed hypospadias with intact prepuce and is uncommon. Often, this is detected once a child has had the foreskin retracted for the first time. As previously mentioned, if this is noticed at the time of circumcision, it is imperative that this should not proceed until the child has been assessed by a paediatric urologist as the foreskin is often used in the operative repair of hypospadias.

The third feature of hypospadias is the most important functionally and that is the downward curve of the penis due to the replacement of the normal corpus spongiosum with scar tissue. This is termed *chordee*, and the correction of this to allow the penis to become straight during erections is an essential component of any surgical repair. It is telling that even the earliest recorded account of hypospadias by Galen recognised this as the most important component of hypospadias resulting in infertility.

The fourth feature of hypospadias is often overlooked on superficial examination. There is often a degree of *penoscrotal transposition*. The uppermost portion of the scrotum comes to lie above the dorsal aspect of the penis, surrounding it in scrotalized skin. This is an important physical finding as it points to a lack of virilisation of the external genitalia in the male. In the most severe cases, it is associated with a bifid scrotum.

The fifth and final component of hypospadias, *urethral hypoplasia*, is often overlooked as there are no obvious physical signs. The male urethra is often hypoplastic in patients with hypospadias. This is often only obvious at the time of attempted hypospadias repair when a seemingly distal hypospadias is actually much more significant once repair is attempted. The distal urethra is often very shallow and small, and in such cases, it is necessary to convert the hypospadias to a more proximal opening before attempting a staged repair.

Assessment of the Infant with Hypospadias

Hypospadias is a relatively common abnormality, being seen in 1:200–300 live births in the United Kingdom. The reported incidence of hypospadias is very wide (3–8:1000) and the incidence appears to be increasing in frequency, although the reason for this is unclear. Once an abnormality of the external genitalia is noted, it is important to complete a thorough assessment of the child with a detailed history and examination.

The majority of cases are spontaneous, although in some families there is a strong family history of hypospadias, familial clustering is seen in around 10% of cases. The recurrence risk in male siblings is 15% and the incidence in fathers of a child with hypospadias is around half of this (7%). A number of different candidate genes have been identified (DAX1, WT1, SOX9) and further evidence for a genetic component is the association of hypospadias in a large number of different syndromes (WAGR syndrome, Denys–Drash syndrome).

In general, male infants with distal hypospadias do not require further investigation unless there are other features suggestive of a disorder of sexual development. The most important of these to recognise is the presence of impalpable gonads in association with hypospadias. A solitary impalpable testis with hypospadias may be the only feature to alert the clinician to the possibility of an abnormality in the sex chromosomes, with sex chromosome mosaicism. Those boys unfortunate enough to have bilateral impalpable gonads require urgent specialist assessment to rule out a more serious disorder of sexual differentiation. It is possible to have normal-looking male external genitalia but to be a virilised 46XX female because of congenital adrenal hyperplasia. Failure to recognise this can be catastrophic, as impaired mineralocorticoid and glucocorticoid synthesis may result in a salt-losing crisis and death. Fortunately, such situations are rare; however, the incidence of congenital adrenal hyperplasia (CAH) is 1:15,000 and so it must be considered in the apparently male infant with impalpable testes.

In cases of proximal hypospadias, it is more important to adequately rule out other significant pathologies. There is some limited evidence that proximal hypospadias is associated with urinary tract abnormalities and a renal tract ultrasound scan can be helpful. The complete assessment of complex genital abnormalities is best done in the context of a multidisciplinary team involving neonatologists, endocrinologists, a paediatric urologist as well as other specialists to perform a timely assessment of gender. This is very important as the incorrect gender label due to an inadequate assessment at birth creates many problems for the child and family in the short, medium and long term.

Surgical Management of Hypospadias

The surgical management of hypospadias is complex. There are a variety of different operations utilised. In distal hypospadias, the two most commonly performed operations are the Mathieu hypospadias repair or a variant of the Snodgrass procedure. These operations traditionally have resulted in the sacrifice of the foreskin to complete a cosmetic repair, although some centres advocate foreskin reconstruction as well. The reported results from the correction of distal hypospadias are excellent with most authors reporting success rates above 85–90%, with minimal long-term complications and excellent cosmetic results. Disappointingly, the literature is much less clear when it comes to examining long-term outcomes in these patients.

More proximal hypospadias can be approached with a wide variety of different techniques, but essentially they fall into staged or single-stage operations. Probably the most commonly used operation is the staged Bracka hypospadias repair, where skin from the inner layer of the foreskin or from inside the mouth is laid on the urethral plate after the removal of the scar tissue and correction of the chordee. This is tubularised as a second-stage operation with the repair of the glans resulting in a circumcised appearance of the penis. Although some authors report very high success rates for these procedures, there are significantly more complications, and the long-term results are not as good as for boys with uncomplicated distal hypospadias.

Following surgical correction, it is important for these boys to be followed up. This is not only to assess the outcomes of the original operation, but also to monitor boys for the development of long-term complications from the surgery. In general, operations for hypospadias are performed at around the age of 1 year, allowing for even staged procedures to be completed by 2 years. Most surgeons place a stent in the urethra following hypospadias repair, and it is easier to do this in young boys as they tolerate this better than boys who have already achieved continence. Following discharge, patients are typically followed up for a minimum of 1 year, and it is this authors' practice to document a normal urine flow rate prior to discharging patients. This is usually possible in boys between the age of 2 and 3 years. It is important that families are given information about the risk of long-term consequences of hypospadias surgery as part of the consent process and are given a list of problems that can occur if they are to be discharged from long-term follow-up. Many surgeons follow up on patients following hypospadias surgery until they leave childhood.

Summary

Hypospadias is a relatively common abnormality of the external genitalia; it has a prevalence of 1:200–300 in the United Kingdom currently, although the incidence seems to be increasing. The early recognition of hypospadias and appropriate referral to specialist centres allows for parents to be given timely and accurate information regarding this condition, although in general the surgical management of patients does not commence until 1 year of age.

It is essential to recognise early those patients with hypospadias as part of a more complex abnormality in sexual differentiation. Practically this means that assessment of the position of the testes at the time of recognition of hypospadias is crucial. When both testes are adequately descended and palpable within a well-developed scrotum, no further investigation is required urgently. However, abnormalities of testicular descent or of scrotal development can point to more serious problems and should be investigated urgently. In general, more complicated cases of hypospadias should be discussed early with tertiary or quaternary centres to allow for appropriate and timely investigations to be performed, and so that parents can be given clear advice.

The operative management of hypospadias is undertaken by specialist surgeons, and the results for distal hypospadias are excellent. Often this can be performed as day case surgery; few patients have long-term complications from surgery. Proximal hypospadias, particularly when in association with either other syndromes or disorders of sexual development, have poorer long-term outcomes. There is no perfect operation for the correction of hypospadias, and long-term data outlining the advantages and disadvantages of different techniques is lacking in the literature.

ACQUIRED ABNORMALITIES OF THE MALE EXTERNAL GENITALIA

The Foreskin

Problems with the foreskin (or prepuce) are common in boys. Whilst there is only limited published literature on the subject, it is clear the author has worked in both temperate and tropical climates that acquired problems with the foreskin, which are encountered more commonly in clinical practice in tropical areas. An audit of cases locally demonstrated a two to three times higher incidence of *balanitis xerotica obliterans* (BXO) in our patients compared to the published figures quoted from other major metropolitan centres, despite this, the incidence of BXO remains relatively uncommon, with an incidence of 1:200–300 in boys under the age of 16. The prepuce plays a role in early childhood to protect the fragile external urethral meatus in the male infant.

It is important to consider that the prepuce is usually non-retractile at birth and becomes retractile without medical intervention in almost all boys by the age of 16. In early childhood, it is not uncommon for boys to have a *physiological phimosis*. As the foreskin is pulled backwards over the glans penis, the inner layer of the prepuce becomes visible (this looks like a rosebud 'flowering') and a physiological constriction ring of shiny tighter skin can be seen proximal to this (see Figure 13.4). This is common in boys up to the age of 5 years, who often report that attempted retraction is uncomfortable. This non-retractability of the foreskin is termed phimosis (Greek for 'muzzling'), which is an appropriate description of the shape of the foreskin when it fails to retract. These boys often have some ballooning of the foreskin on voiding which is usually entirely benign.

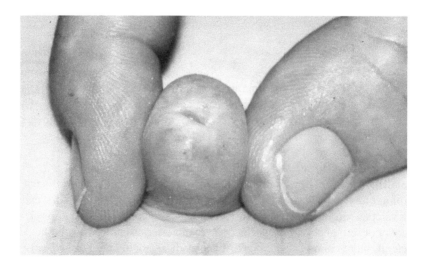

FIGURE 13.4 Balanitis xerotica obliterans (BXO).

In boys who develop a phimosis, subsequent to it having been retractile or in whom the foreskin looks abnormal or scarred on attempted retraction, it is important to consider the possibility of a *pathological phimosis*. In such cases, the preputial orifice becomes cicatrised, leading to a 'shark's mouth' appearance; this almost always occurs only in boys over the age of 5 years. Boys with pathological phimosis may present with difficulty or pain during micturition or may be entirely asymptomatic. There is usually a characteristic pallor, scarring and stenosis of the prepuce. They almost invariably have an abnormal uroflowmetry if this can be performed. The histological appearances of this condition are termed *balanitis xerotica obliterans* (BXO). The condition is unfortunately progressive, ultimately leading to scarring of the glans and urethra and so early referral and assessment is important if this condition is suspected. BXO remains relatively uncommon, affecting only around 1:500–800 uncircumcised boys under the age of 16 years. An example of a case of BXO can be seen in Figure 13.4.

It is not uncommon for boys to have problems with recurrent infections or more commonly to complain of redness, soreness and irritation of the foreskin. These episodes are often self-limiting and improve as children get older. They often are treated with oral antibiotics, but it is probably more important to encourage fluid intake, as concentrated urine often exacerbates or initiates episodes of balanitis. It is important to differentiate this from much rarer episodes where the shaft of the penis becomes infected, and these patients should be referred and assessed in a secondary care setting as often intravenous antibiotics are required.

The relative merits of circumcision are beyond the scope of this chapter, but it is important to consider the risks vs the benefits of circumcision which change as children pass through childhood and adolescence. The natural history of the majority of benign pathologies of the foreskin is to improve as children get older, particularly as they pass through puberty. A *paraphimosis* is a condition where the foreskin retracts backwards over the glans penis and cannot be drawn forward again getting stuck on the coronal sulcus. This condition is distressing and often embarrassing for the child which may result in delayed presentation. Fortunately, it is uncommon but requires urgent treatment and assessment in secondary care and almost always it is wise to circumcise young men after such an event.

It is important to remember that there are rare congenital abnormalities of the foreskin (for example, a hooded foreskin/congenital megaprepuce), which should be assessed by a paediatric urologist. The management of acute testicular pain and common and inguinoscrotal pathologies are discussed elsewhere.

PROBLEMS OF THE EXTERNAL GENITALIA IN GIRLS

Congenital Problems of the Female External Genitalia

Unlike in the male infant, it is uncommon to identify problems with the external genitalia in a female. An understanding of the complex nature of normal sexual differentiation described earlier helps to explain when and why problems can occur. The commonest disorder of sexual differentiation is the virilised 46XX female, which accounts for 85% of all cases of female neonates born with ambiguous genitalia. The incidence is approximately 1:15,000 live births.

Congenital Adrenal Hyperplasia

CAH is a consequence of the failure of the normal metabolic pathways involved in steroid hormone biosynthesis. Failure to be able to form cortisol results in failure of the normal negative feedback to produce adrenocorticotropic hormone (ACTH) and subsequently an overproduction of cortisol precursors which result in inappropriate virilisation of the female neonate.

The management of ambiguous genitalia is complex and requires urgent input from neonatal/paediatric endocrine and paediatric urology teams as life-threatening salt wasting can occur early in neonatal life.

Imperforate Hymen

A small number of girls are born with an imperforate hymen. Clinically this presents as a bulging introital mass in a neonatal girl, or less commonly as primary amenorrhoea or urinary retention in the pubertal girl. It is possible to detect vaginal distention antenatally during routine antenatal scans and this is an increasingly frequent mode of presentation. The treatment is surgical incision of the imperforate hymen to allow the normal flow of menses to be established during puberty.

Vaginal Agenesis (Mayer–Rokitansky Syndrome)

This can occur as an isolated abnormality but is mostly seen as part of a spectrum of abnormalities resulting from a failure of organogenesis of the mesonephric and paramesonephric duct structures. In Mayer–Rokitansky syndrome, the upper two-thirds of the vagina is absent, but the vagina may be completely absent or there may simply be a dimple in the perineum. This condition is the most common cause of primary amenorrhoea.

Cloacal Anomalies

Cloacal deformities are rare and occur in about 1 in 20,000–25,000 newborn females. These rare malformations are a form of congenital anorectal malformation. In a cloacal deformity, the rectum, vagina and urethra structures join into one common channel. There is only one opening visible on the perineum at birth (see Figure 13.5). These patients require urgent referral and assessment by a

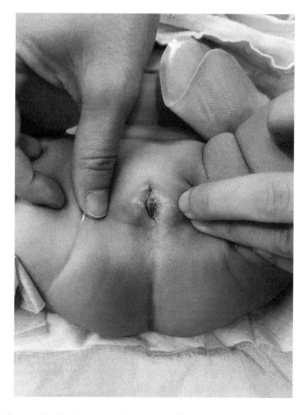

FIGURE 13.5   Female infant with single perineal opening (cloaca).

paediatric urologist. Cloacal deformities are classified depending on where these three tracts merge. If the common channel is short, then often there is no immediate low obstruction to either the urinary or gastrointestinal tract. If the common channel is longer, then patients can present with intestinal obstruction.

ACQUIRED ABNORMALITIES IN GIRLS

Acquired problems with the female external genitalia are seen much more commonly than congenital conditions.

Labial Adhesions

Parents often present with concerns surrounding an abnormal appearance of the external genitalia. This is often due to the wide range of normal appearances of the external genitalia in the female; however, the most frequent problem is labial adhesions where the labia minora become fused together resulting in a 'blank' appearance to the perineum (see Figure 13.6). These are most commonly present in girls between the ages of 2 and 6 and are thought to be a response to episodes of inflammation (vulvovaginitis). They rarely cause problems requiring medical intervention but occasionally can cause obstruction or deviation in the normal urinary stream. In the worst cases, this can even result in girls finding it difficult to keep the diverted flow of urine into the toilet or potty during toilet training or voiding, as the urinary stream may be directed upwards by dense labial adhesions; in such cases, surgical division is often required. In most cases, labial adhesions are entirely asymptomatic and do not require treatment.

The natural history of labial adhesions is that they resolve spontaneously, and they can be managed conservatively. Surgical separation or therapy with oestrogen creams has been tried, but in prepubertal girls, the lack of circulating oestrogens means that they often reform after discontinuation of the topical oestrogen cream. Parental reassurance and patient watchful waiting is usually all that is required.

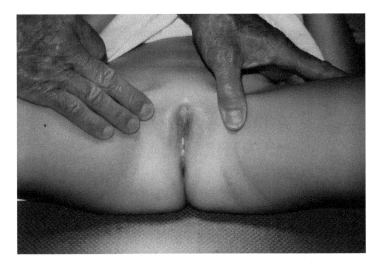

FIGURE 13.6   Labial adhesions.

Vaginal Discharge

Vulvovaginitis is relatively common in prepubertal girls, but vaginal discharge is uncommon. There is a wide differential diagnosis, but if persistent or severe, it is important to rule out serious underlying pathology. It is important to consider a retained vaginal foreign body from a small item, such as a small toy or Lego brick, placed in the vagina and forgotten about, although this is rare. Other pathologies include bacterial infections (including sexually transmitted infections), sexual abuse and genitourinary malignancies (vaginal rhabdomyosarcoma), but these are rare. If sexual abuse is considered, the child protection team should be consulted.

After taking a careful history and completing a physical examination, then a pelvic ultrasound scan can be a useful first-line investigation. Microbiology swabs may identify causative organisms, which may include *Neisseria gonorrhoeae* in the case of sexual abuse. Examination under anaesthesia, including cystoscopy and vaginoscopy, may ultimately be necessary and may also be therapeutic in the case of vaginal foreign bodies.

Vaginal Bleeding

Vulvovaginitis may be associated with occasional 'spotting' of blood on the undergarments; however, frank vaginal bleeding is rare and can be the presenting sign of serious underlying disease. Vaginal rhabdomyosarcoma, although rare, is the most important potential diagnosis to exclude. It is much less common than trauma and foreign bodies. Other causes include vascular malformations, precocious puberty and sexual abuse. An ultrasound of the pelvis with skilled hands can be helpful, but an examination under anaesthesia may be required.

SUMMARY

- Problems with the genitalia are more common in boys than in girls.
- Testicular maldescent is the most common problem requiring surgery.
- Foreskin problems are mostly benign, but it is important to recognise pathological phimosis.
- Suspected disorders of sexual differentiation require immediate referral to a specialist centre for multidisciplinary care.
- Acquired problems are much more common in girls than congenital problems.

FURTHER READING

Abdelrahman HM, Feloney MP. Imperforate hymen. In: StatPearls [Internet]. Treasure Island (FL): StatPearls Publishing; 2022.

Anderson J, Paterek E. Vaginal foreign body evaluation and treatment. In: StatPearls [Internet]. Treasure Island (FL): StatPearls Publishing; 2022.

Celis S, Reed F, Murphy F, Adams S, Gillick J, Abdelhafeez AH, Lopez PJ. Balanitis xerotica obliterans in children and adolescents: A literature review and clinical series. J Pediatr Urol. 2014 February;10(1):34–9.

El-Maouche D, Arlt W, Merke DP. Congenital adrenal hyperplasia. Lancet. 2017 November;390(10108):2194–210.

Gluckman S, Karpelowsky J, Webster AC, McGee RG. Management for intussusception in children. Cochrane Database Syst Rev. 2017 June;6(6):CD006476.

Gurney JK, McGlynn KA, Stanley J, Merriman T, Signal V, Shaw C, Edwards R, Richiardi L, Hutson J, Sarfati D. Risk factors for cryptorchidism. Nat Rev Urol. 2017 September;14(9):534–48. doi: 10.1038/nrurol.2017.90.

Hutson JM. Cryptorchidism and hypospadias. 2018 Jul (10). In: Feingold KR, Anawalt B, Boyce A, Chrousos G, de Herder WW, Dhatariya K, Dungan K, Hershman JM, Hofland J, Kalra S, Kaltsas G, Koch C, Kopp P, Korbonits M, Kovacs CS, Kuohung W, Laferrère B, Levy M, McGee EA, McLachlan R, Morley JE, New M, Purnell J, Sahay R, Singer F, Sperling MA, Stratakis CA, Trence DL, Wilson DP, editors. Endotext [Internet]. South Dartmouth (MA): MDText.com, Inc.; 2000.

Romano ME. Prepubertal vulvovaginitis. Clin Obstet Gynecol. 2020 September;63(3):479–85.

Snodgrass WT. Snodgrass technique for hypospadias repair. BJU Int. 2005 March;95(4):683–93.

Minimally Invasive Paediatric Surgery

14

David Kanaganayangam and Bhanu
Mariyappa Rathnamma

INTRODUCTION

Traditional surgical techniques involve large incision to provide the surgeon with ample views and space to physically handle the required organ. Advances in technologies in recent decades have stimulated radical changes to the approach of surgical procedures towards minimally invasive surgical techniques. In essence, this involves the insertion of a scope into a body cavity via a small incision or natural orifice and further insertion of instruments by other smaller incisions. Minimally invasive techniques offer potential benefits to the patients and healthcare systems, including reduced postoperative pain, shorter lengths of stay in hospital, quicker return to schooling and better cosmesis.

Keeling performed the first laparoscopic procedure in Germany in 1901 using a rigid cystoscope in an animal model and Jacobaeus published the first human series within the decade. These initial procedures were primarily diagnostic with the first therapeutic procedure being described in the 1930s by Fevers who performed an abdominal adhesiolysis with the laparoscope. The development of fibre optic technology and its incorporation with the scope in 1954 by Hopkins dramatically improved both illumination and image quality. The first laparoscopic appendicectomy was performed in the 1970s and laparoscopic cholecystectomy within a decade.

By the late 1990s, the laparoscopic approach to cholecystectomies had become the standard of care in developed countries and applications of minimally invasive surgery had been found in the majority of surgical specialities.

While the introduction of minimally invasive techniques to paediatric surgery was more reserved in comparison to adult surgery, there has been a rapid rise in the number of paediatric procedures being performed via minimally invasive techniques. The current evidence base of minimally invasive paediatric surgery is growing with applications in thoracic, gastrointestinal, urological and neonatal procedures.

While minimally invasive techniques bring novel approaches to surgical procedures, they are accompanied by the challenges of requiring new skills by surgeons and operative team. The novelty of tools, psychomotor skills, equipment and vantages of anatomical landmarks means that there is a substantial learning curve associated with the utilisation of minimally invasive techniques. As such, training is a fundamental aspect of implementing safe techniques. Early studies of many minimally invasive techniques demonstrated high incidences of complications in comparison to current complication rates.

DOI: 10.1201/9781003156659-14

GENERAL PRINCIPLES OF LAPAROSCOPIC SURGERY

The aim of minimally invasive surgery safely performs a procedure while causing the least amount of anatomical, physiological and psychological trauma to the patient. This is generally achieved through the use of scopes into body cavities through a small incision to visualise the operative field with further small incisions to accommodate instruments.

Advantages

- Small incisions
- Less postoperative pain
- Reduced wound-related complications such as infection for herniations
- Decreased tissue trauma
- Decreased physiological effect
- Earlier return to full activity
- Shorter hospital stays with improved cost effectiveness
- Improved visualisation of the operative field
- Improved training/teaching

Disadvantages

- Loss of tactile feedback from tissues
- Potential difficulty in controlling major bleeding with loss of visual field
- Longer procedure times
- Requirement for specialised skill set
- Requirement of specialised instruments
- Increased risk of iatrogenic injuries for disorientation of anatomy or unrecognised "out of site" injuries

CHOICE OF INSUFFLATING GASES

Multiple gases have been trialled for insufflation in laparoscopic and thoracoscopic surgery. The ideal gas for insufflation would be an inert, non-flammable, colourless gas with a high tissue permeability, blood solubility and capable of undergoing pulmonary excretion. Other considerations include cost, access and potential to cause side effects.

Carbon dioxide has become the insufflation gas of choice for laparoscopy as it is colourless and has a high blood solubility, reducing the risk of air embolus compared to other gases. It is also easily assessable and inexpensive. It does, however, have the potential to cause several side effects. These include hypercapnia, respiratory acidosis and cardiac dysrhythmias. Carbon dioxide also causes more of an inflammatory response in the tissues compared with other gases, resulting in increased postoperative pain from diaphragmatic and peritoneal irritation.

Nitrous oxide causes less peritoneal irritation and decreased risk of dysrhythmias compared with carbon dioxide. However, it does have the disadvantages of causing decreased blood pressure and has the potential for combustion in the presence of hydrogen or methane. Air similarly supports combustion and has a high risk of gas embolus compared with CO_2. Helium is inert, however, has the highest risk of gas embolus. Oxygen is not used as it if highly combustible.

PHYSIOLOGICAL EFFECTS OF PNEUMOPERITONEUM

Increased intra-abdominal pressure (IAP) from the insufflation displaces the diaphragm cranially and decreased pulmonary compliance. This reduces the functional residual capacity of the lungs and causes atelectasis and intrapulmonary shunting, promoting hypoxaemia. Pulmonary compliance is also reduced with increased peak airway pressures.

Increased IAP from the pneumoperitoneum can cause vascular compression and increase systemic peripheral vascular resistance. The resulting increased afterload with decreased preload, together, decreased cardiac output. Decreased mean arterial pressure (MAP) and increased in IAP reduce the abdominal perfusion pressure. The first sign of decreased intra-abdominal perfusion is decreased urine output from renal hypoperfusion.

Ergonomics

While minimally invasive surgery aims to decrease the trauma of surgery to the patient, these techniques can be more physically demanding on the surgeons. Ergonomical set-up of the operating theatre and surgical access approach significantly improve the surgeon's experience and reduces complications.

Port placement: The "baseball diamond" port placement is a concept to describe the ergonomic placement of laparoscopic port. With the operative target at the second base position, the optical port is placed at the home base position with left and right working ports at the third and first base positions, respectively. This facilitates optimal triangulation of the instruments and depth perception. In-line visualisation describes the placement of monitor in line with the operative target. This aligns the surgeon's visual and motor axis through the operation.

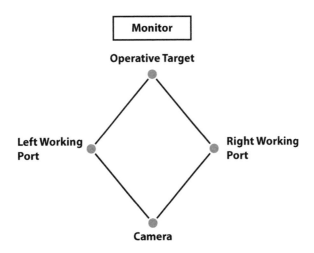

Laparoscopic instruments function as a lever with the fulcrum at the level of abdominal wall. The ports should be placed to facilitate equal length of instruments intra-abdominally and externally. This creates a type 1 lever, where the force applied by the surgeon externally equates to the force exerted on the tissue. Having a greater length intra-abdominally amplifies with force on the operative target.

APPLYING MIS TECHNIQUES TO PAEDIATRIC POPULATIONS

There are several challenges in applying minimally invasive techniques to the paediatric patient which contributed to the slower uptake by paediatric surgeons. Most notably being the smaller size of the patients and relatively larger liver and intra-abdominal bladder. With minimally invasive techniques already being significantly more technically challenging than the open operations, the decreased operative space further amplifies the complexity. Smaller surface areas result in increased risk of instrument clashing and suboptimal triangulation. Similarly, the ergonomics of operating within small spaces requires variations to the equipment. Equal intra- and extracorporeal lengths of the instruments optimise the ergonomics of procedure. Use of instruments which are both shorter and thinner (2–3 mm diameter) is required for the small paediatric patients.

Smaller diameter scopes have reduced light transmission; however, with improving technology, suitable image quality is now easily obtainable with small scopes. The use of wider angle lenses/displays optimises views in the small operative field.

There are several physiological factors that make abdominal insufflation in laparoscopic surgery potentially more hazardous in the paediatric patient. Children have predominantly diaphragmatic respirations, with increased chest wall compliance and rate-dependent cardiac output. Children are also more likely to have right to left cardiac shunts. Concurrent respiratory disease, particularly in the neonatal patients, may exacerbate pulmonary complications of overinsufflation. Children have more compliant abdominal wall, and as such, lower inflation pressures are required to achieve optimal working space. Infants typically require pressures of 8–10 mmHg, with children 2–10 years of age requiring 10–12 mmHg and older children requiring 15 mmHg.

APPLICATIONS OF MIS

Abdominal Surgery

Being one of the most common surgical pathologies in childhood, the laparoscopic appendicectomy was one of the first minimally invasive techniques to be commonly utilised by paediatric surgeons. A major advantage of the laparoscopic approach in comparison to the standard open appendicectomy is the diagnostic capacity of the procedure. With the differentials for abdominal pain being broad in the paediatric patient, laparoscopy allows for easy inspection of intra-abdominal and pelvic organs.

Gastro-oesophageal reflux disease (GORD) is a common condition affecting the paediatric population. While the majority of children with GORD have spontaneous resolution of symptoms, in some children with persistent symptoms and complications refractory to lifestyle and pharmacological therapies, surgical management is indicated. Laparoscopic anti-reflux procedures such as the Nissen fundoplication have shown to have similar efficacy to open operations with reduced complications in children.

Treatment of infantile pyloric stenosis requires surgical division of muscle fibres of the pylorus, pyloromyotomy. Both open and laparoscopic approaches are commonly using in clinical practice. Randomised controlled trials comparing the approaches have demonstrated equivalent outcomes with statistically significant reduction in length of stay and time to resumption of feeding with laparoscopic approach.

Inguinal hernia repair is one of the most common paediatric surgical procedures performed. Several techniques have been described to laparoscopically approach the repair. Benefits include easy visual assessment for contralateral hernias. A recent meta-analysis suggests no clinical improvement of outcomes of laparoscopic versus an open approach; however, further high-quality prospective studies are needed to further compare.

Biliary reconstructive surgery for choledochal cysts or biliary atresia has traditionally been performed via a generous muscle dissecting laparotomy to create a portoenterostomy (Kasai procedure) or hepaticojejunostomy, respectively. Laparoscopic approaches to these reconstructions have proven to be feasible and effective in paediatric populations. Despite this, the required laparoscopic dissection, suturing and knot tying have meant that these are technically challenging procedures with a substantial learning curve. Recent applications of robotic-assisted biliary reconstructions, with three-dimensional images and articulated instruments, have shown address some of these challenges.

Outside the setting of trauma, splenectomies are often indicated for haematological conditions such as hereditary spherocytosis or idiopathic thrombocytopenia. These conditions are often associated with splenomegaly and potentially symptomatic cholelithiasis. Laparoscopic approaches to splenectomy have proven to be safe and effective despite significant splenomegaly. Additionally, a laparoscopic approach facilitates concurrent cholecystectomy. Laparoscopic approach result is decreased length of hospital stay and postoperative pain.

Laparoscopy has also been utilised in assessment in paediatric trauma, management of inflammatory bowel disease, assessment of gastrointestinal bleeding, adrenalectomies and distal pancreatectomies for malignancies. With increasing incidence of childhood obesity, bariatric surgery in adolescent patients has demonstrated similar outcomes to resolutions of co-morbidities and sustainable weight loss in comparison to adults.

Urological

Laparoscopy is a key tool in the assessment and management of impalpable testis. Firstly, it can be used to identify the absence of testis or locate an intra-abdominal testicle. In the latter, a two-stage Fowler-Stephens orchidopexy is the standard approach. In the first stage, the testicular vessels are divided to allow collateralisation of blood supply to occur. In the second stage, either via an inguinal or laparoscopic approach, the testicle is mobilised into the scrotum.

Non-functioning kidneys are often atrophic and cystic. As such, a nephrectomy can be carried out via a minimally invasive approach without the need for a large incision for removal of the specimen. Transperitoneal and retroperitoneal laparoscopic approaches have proven to demonstrate reduced post-surgical pain and length of stay. Transperitoneal and retroperitoneal laparoscopic approaches to pyeloplasty for pelvi-ureteric junction dysfunction have been performed with comparable outcomes to standard open approach. This is a technically challenging procedure requiring laparoscopic suture anastomosis, especially in the infant patient with narrow ureter. Similar to biliary reconstructions, robotic surgery has shown to benefit in addressing some of these challenges.

Neonatal Laparoscopic Surgery

Minimally invasive techniques have a role in the management of several neonatal conditions. Intestinal atresia can be assessed and repaired laparoscopically. In Hirschsprung's disease laparoscopic biopsies can be taken to assess the level of ganglionosis and the bowel can be laparoscopically mobilised for the anorectal pull through procedure. Similarly, in children with anorectal malformations, laparoscopy can be beneficial in identifying the location of fistulae.

Open surgical repair of oesophageal atresia and tracheo-oesophageal fistula is one of the most technically challenging procedures in paediatric surgery. The first thoracoscopically repair was reported in 1999; however, minimally invasive techniques are not commonly used. Studies have demonstrated the safety and efficacy of the thoracoscopic approach comparable to open thoracotomy. However, there is limited evidence of long-term outcomes between the two techniques.

Congenital diaphragmatic hernia repairs in the neonatal period have been reported via both laparoscopic and thoracoscopic approaches with good outcomes. Associated pulmonary hypoplasia and pulmonary hypertension need to be considered in the selection of these neonates for minimally invasive approaches and further prospective trials are needed to better compare techniques.

Thoracoscopic Surgery in Children

Musculoskeletal deformity and shoulder dysfunction are common sequelae of traditional thoracotomy, especially in the growing child. Video-assisted thoracoscopic surgery (VATS) with single lung ventilation has become a major thoracic approach for paediatric surgeons for numerous indications.

In addition to oesophageal atresia/tracheo-oesophageal fistula and congenital diaphragmatic hernia repairs mentioned earlier, VATS has been utilised for the management of empyema's and pulmonary resection. VATS and decortication for empyema is generally a second-line option following drainage and urokinase; however, there has been some support for its earlier use.

Thoracoscopic resection of congenital and acquired lung lesions had shown to be as safe and effective as open procedures and has the advantages of reduced postoperative pain and length of stay.

Other thoracoscopic procedures reported include aortopexy for severe tracheomalacia, pectus excavatum repair and ligation of symptomatic patent ductus arteriosus.

FUTURE DEVELOPMENT AND ADVANCING TECHNOLOGIES

As the technologies continue to evolve and the evidence base grows, innovation in minimally invasive paediatric surgery will likely continue to progress and techniques be modified.

Robotic surgery allows better articulation of instruments, stabilisation and three-dimensional visualisation of the operative field, addressing technical challenges of standard laparoscopy. As access to robotic surgery improves, application of these techniques will broaden what is achievable with minimally invasive techniques.

Advances in digitisation and augmentation of surgery allow surgeons to access additional information intraoperatively. This can incorporate imaging-guided surgery with access to preoperative and intraoperative imaging to assist in decision-making. Videoconferencing allows input from consultant specialist in real-time assessment and decision-making. Augmented-reality-assisted surgery is being applied to provide intra-operative navigation utilising computer-generated reconstruction from preoperative imaging and overlaying descriptive imaging onto the operative display. Another area or potential advancement is the use of artificial intelligence algorithms to process intra-operative data and provide real-time feedback to surgeons.

CONCLUSION AND SUMMARY

Minimally invasive surgical techniques have a central role in paediatric surgery with utilisation in all areas of the speciality, having become the standard of care in several conditions. minimally invasive surgery (MIS) techniques improve postoperative pain, shortened hospital stays and quick return to activity. As the evidence base and innovation continue to evolve, the role of MIS is likely to continue to grow in paediatric surgery.

FURTHER READING

Blinman T, Ponsky T. Pediatric minimally invasive surgery: Laparoscopy and thoracoscopy in infants and children. Pediatrics. 2012 September;130(3):539–49.

Holcomb GW 3rd. Thoracoscopic surgery for esophageal atresia. Pediatr Surg Int. 2017 April;33(4):475–81.

Mei H, Pu J, Yang C, Zhang H, Zheng L, Tong Q. Laparoscopic versus open pyeloplasty for ureteropelvic junction obstruction in children: A systematic review and meta-analysis. J Endourol. 2011 May;25(5):727–36.

Meinzer A, Alkatout I, Krebs TF, Baastrup J, Reischig K, Meiksans R, Bergholz R. Advances and trends in pediatric minimally invasive surgery. J Clin Med. 2020 December;9(12):3999.

Redden MD, Chin TY, van Driel ML. Surgical versus non-surgical management for pleural empyema. Cochrane Database Syst Rev. 2017 March;3(3):CD010651.

Ru W, Wu P, Feng S, Lai XH, Chen G. Laparoscopic versus open Nissen fundoplication in children: A systematic review and meta-analysis. J Pediatr Surg. 2016 October;51(10):1731–6.

Steyaert H, Valla JS. Minimally invasive urologic surgery in children: An overview of what can be done. Eur J Pediatr Surg. 2005 October;15(5):307–13.

Global Health Interventions in Paediatric Surgery

15

Ramesh Mark Nataraja, Yin Mar Oo and Elizabeth McLeod

INTRODUCTION

There has been a shift in the focus of global health initiatives in recent years. In the past, there was a targeted approach to programmes that focussed on outcomes such as surveillance and control of infectious diseases, including vaccinations, health or traditional education, health promotion and disease prevention. However, although these remain a priority in low-resource settings, there is now an increasing interest in the provision of safe and affordable surgical care in low- and middle-income countries (LMICs). This has been driven by the estimate that there are more than 5 billion people worldwide who have a deficit in their access to safe and affordable surgical care and of these 1.7 billion are either children or adolescents. The COVID-19 pandemic has highlighted global inequity with access to vaccines, and the same applies to access to surgical and maternal healthcare services. There is also an increasing evidence based on the cost-effectiveness analysis (CEA) for medical interventions and system-wide analysis in LMICs has revealed that surgery can be a cost-effective intervention.

Simulation-based education (SBE) is well established in many high-income countries (HICs). SBE may be regarded as the gold standard for healthcare professional education, for medical and nursing curricula, in terms of knowledge, skills and behaviour acquisition which improve patient-related outcomes. There are many different modalities of SBE, which allow the healthcare provider to achieve competency utilising mastery learning and deliberate practice in a safe environment prior to patient contact. Limitations to the application and effectiveness of SBE in LMICs are reported; however, our organisation has partnered with clinician colleagues in low-resource settings to apply SBE with proven clinical results.

In this chapter, we will focus primarily on SBE and faculty capacity development as these are relatively novel compared with more traditional service delivery interventions.

MONASH CHILDREN'S SIMULATION EXPERIENCE

For over 5 years, Monash Children's Simulation (MCS), in partnership with other organisations such as Monash Children's Hospital International (MCHI), the Royal Australasian College of Surgeons (RACS) and the Department of Foreign Affairs and Trade, has been delivering various educational activities in LMICs. The MCHI/MCS Myanmar programme is described in Figure 15.1.

DOI: 10.1201/9781003156659-15

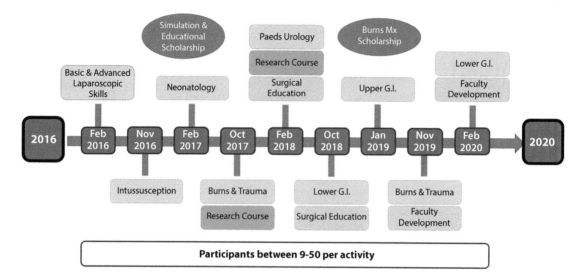

FIGURE 15.1 Overview of the MCHI/MCS Myanmar programme.

Application of Simulation-Based Education to a LMIC

Simulation-based education is often perceived as requiring significant funding and resources to deliver effective educational activities, which may therefore render it an inappropriate modality in LMICs. In high-resource settings, SBE is often delivered in purpose-built simulation centres using expensive equipment such as high-technology mannequins and part task trainers, which compounds this perception. Cost reporting is often infrequent or incomplete in SBE research, which also limits its uptake in low-resource settings. However, it is vital to first consider the specific educational objectives and desired outcomes of the activity rather than the available equipment. The fidelity of an educational activity or its functional task alignment is related to whether it confers the competency or skill that is intended, and therefore cost should not be an initial consideration. For example, if the intended educational outcome is to acquire competency with endotracheal intubation, this may not only be performed on a high-technology mannequin, but competency could also be achieved with a low-cost bench trainer. This also has the added benefits of minimal maintenance requirements. Therefore, with the design of an educational activity, the first step is the determination what needs to be taught, the learning objectives, followed by the most appropriate educational tool to achieve this in a particular context.

Laparoscopic Simulation-Based Education

There have been significant technological advances in recent years that allow laparoscopic bench trainers to be applied to all settings. An example of this includes the eoSim™ box-trainer simulator (eoSurgical, UK) with a tablet as the video source and a portable battery as a light source. As these portable laparoscopic simulators collapse down into a briefcase-type container, they can be easily transported anywhere in the world. This facilitates the creation of portable surgical simulation centres as we have used in the MCHI/MCS Myanmar programme. These simulators can then be combined with a variety of different validated laparoscopic tasks such as the double glove or eoSim core tasks to enable the acquisition of laparoscopic skills in any setting. As for any SBE programme, these low-cost simulators should be available outside of the confines of educational courses, to allow deliberate and self-directed practice. Other successful programmes such as the Fundamentals of Laparoscopic Surgery (FLS®) can also be applied with

TABLE 15.1   Key potential advantages of laparoscopic surgery in a LMIC

	ADVANTAGES OF LAPAROSCOPY IN A LMIC

Clinical	1. Shortened hospital length of stay, decreased pain and faster return to work
	2. Improved clinical outcomes:
	   a. Smaller wounds in a potentially unclean water supply setting
	   b. Decreased infections
	   c. Fewer long-term complications (incisional hernias and adhesions)
	   d. Less immunosuppression
	   e. Less abdominal drainage
	3. Decreased unnecessary appendectomies
	4. Reduction in unnecessary laparotomies in the setting of limited cross-sectional imaging and other diagnostic methods for various conditions (tuberculosis, intra-abdominal malignancies, pelvic inflammatory disease, trauma)
	5. Potentially diagnostic and therapeutic for certain conditions (Ascariasis in the biliary tree and gynaecological pathology)

Economic	1. Equipment cost ratio for laparoscopy/ultrasound/CT/MRI is 1:500:2500:4500 2. Minimal use of analgesia, antibiotics, intravenous fluid therapy and other medical supplies 3. Earlier discharge from hospital 4. Individual patient advantages of lower hospital bill and quicker return to work
Systemic	1. Increased availability of hospital beds for other patients 2. Coupled with a laparoscopic training programme also facilitates courses for basic and emergency surgical services 3. Increased confidence in the local health system

these benchtop simulators as they have been in low-resource setting in Africa. As with any educational activity, the provision of feedback is crucial for meaningful long-term changes in learner behaviours and practice, which in the future may be provided by telementoring.

Laparoscopic simulation is a potentially controversial topic when discussing educational interventions in low-resource settings. Slow uptake of laparoscopy in LMICs is largely cost driven but there is some evidence that there may be additional barriers. These may include ongoing organisational funding structures rather than initial upfront costs, and a hierarchical local surgical culture, and the expertise and skills associated with a change in practice which may limit the willingness to embrace novel techniques.

The clear advantages of the utilisation of laparoscopy in a LMIC setting are elucidated in the systematic review by Chao et al. (Table 15.1). There is also increasing evidence of the cost-effectiveness of surgical interventions in LMICs, and the initial investment required for laparoscopic surgery may be balanced with decreased requirements for cross-sectional imaging. The introduction of laparoscopy in HICs predated the utilisation of SBE, and a high incidence of bile duct injuries following laparoscopic cholecystectomy reflected the initial learning curve for this operative modality. However, this incidence has now normalised in a HIC setting.

There are various established laparoscopic training programmes, including FLS® which can be adapted for local context and educational requirements in collaboration with local educators.

Laparoscopic SBE is only one aspect of a SBE programme in an LMIC. It should be coupled with the provision of other modalities such as scenario-based, low-cost part task trainers for essential procedural tasks such as endotracheal intubation and basic surgical skills.

Scenario-Based Exercise (SBE)

SBE is one of the most recognised forms of simulation in HICs and forms the foundation of well-recognised courses such as the advanced trauma life support (ATLS©), Emergency Management of

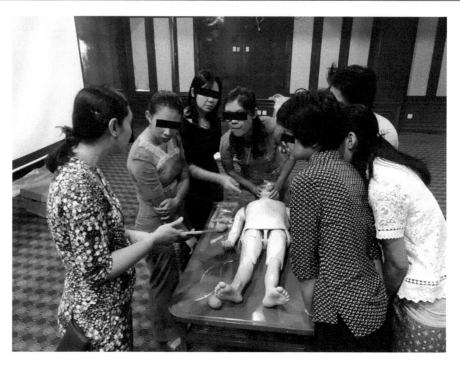

FIGURE 15.2   Senior faculty member at Yangon Children's Hospital delivering a trauma scenario with a low-cost simulator and a tablet for the provision of radiographs and other clinical props.

Severe Burns (EMSB) and Advanced Paediatric Life Support (APLS©). In this SBE modality, a mannequin or other part task trainer is utilised to provide a focus for the activity. In a simulation centre in a HIC setting, this will be a high-technology or "high-fidelity" mannequin; however, this is not usually required to achieve the same educational objectives. For example, if the learning objective of the scenario is to ensure adequate adherence to the ATLS algorithm for the management of a patient with acute trauma, a low-technology basic life support mannequin will be sufficient rather than a high-technology one such as Sim Man (Laerdal™). These activities may be conducted in a clinical space or dedicated educational space, or any space that is available and easily accessible. As there is often a conflict between the need for provision of clinical services and attending educational activities, having these within clinical institutions can be very effective. The importance of including these types of SBE includes the development of cognitive and professional skills such as communication, leadership, teamwork, crisis management and situational awareness. These have all been shown to have a more significant impact on patient safety and outcomes than technical skills alone. SBE also facilitates the development of multi-disciplinary team working skills that may overcome some of the barriers to improve patient care. Once the local faculty has been upskilled to facilitate the activity, there should be a planned transition to conducting the activity in the local language (Figure 15.2).

Basic Surgical Skills

Basic surgical skills have formed a core component of surgical training in both high- and low-resource settings. There are various well-established courses that include the Australia and New Zealand Surgical Skills Education and Training course (ASSET, RACS) and the Basic Surgical Skills course (BSS, Royal College of Surgeons of England). The RCS BSS course, which is part of the mandatory surgical training programme in the United Kingdom, has been utilised in many different country settings, including

Africa and Southeast Asia. This type of core surgical skills training can include the use of hybrid simulation, and either synthetic, cadaveric or animal models to simulate part or the whole of a particular intervention or procedure. Simulators used in these educational activities do not have to be expensive, for example a hand-tying simulator may involve hooks placed onto a wooden board base. Cultural considerations for the use of animal tissue should be carefully considered, including their storage and disposal in a tropical climate. Acknowledgement of an existing high surgical skill level for local faculty in these domains is vital, and they should be included early in all aspects of an SBE programme. Resources that may be lacking, for example suture material, should be anticipated and sourced prior to the activity. Sustainability of supply may be facilitated by fostering relationships with commercial partners and HIC institutions.

Local Needs Assessment and Partnership Building

One of the more frequently applied models that have been applied to interventions in a low-resource setting has been a focus on what can be offered by the visiting team rather than what is needed. This is often done with the experience of success in a different low-resource setting by this visiting team, but as with many aspects of Global Surgery needs assessment should be initially performed with subsequent adaptation to the cultural setting and requirements.

This is especially true when there are multiple teams from different countries visiting at different times and there is a need for co-ordination and maximisation of impact. However, this is not limited to Global Surgery, and it is acknowledged that the health needs of disadvantaged communities in the setting of LMICs are often dictated by data that is often not relevant to the community itself.

For interventions to be effective and have long-term meaningful results require partnership with academic and clinical champions in the LMIC is essential.

The formation of global health partnerships involves potentially complex relationships between the individual clinicians or educators and organisations and both parties have distinct positions, context, needs, resources and agendas. With an increasing realisation of the importance of equity in global health, there are various tools that have been developed to improve this vital component of global health and surgery. Partnerships between HIC and LMIC organisations may have complex issues of power imbalances that are based in complex socio-political and economic histories.

There are many examples of where this can be effective such as the Pacific Islands Project (PIP) with the RACS. This is vital for capacity building which is relevant for the development of an *in country* surgical workforce for the LMIC. The development of a memorandum of understanding (MOU) is a key step in the formation of a long-term relationship, but this will require the initial development of a working relationship based on mutual trust and alignment of objectives and outcomes.

One model that can facilitate this is the incorporation of a faculty debrief at the end of the educational activity. In this, the relevance of the educational content or delivery can be discussed and planning for future interventions. In the MCHI/MCS Myanmar programme, the intussusception of SBE intervention originated from, such as discussion, centring on the management of common paediatric surgical conditions. During these discussions, it became apparent that most of infants with this condition required an operative intervention hence the requirement for the introduction of the air enema technique.

In clinical interventions in Global Surgery including the provision of operative interventions, the impact of the visiting NGO teams should be considered. Often the visiting surgical team will require an operating theatre which will impact negatively on the ability of the local surgeons to provide elective services. This can be overcome with established interventions such as Mercy Ships where all the essential facilities to provide specialist surgical care are transported to the LMIC. However, this is not the case in the majority in NGO interventions. This impact on the provision of surgical care by the local LMIC surgeons is also true for educational interventions. For surgeons to attend these sessions, they must be taken away from providing clinical care and this needs to be incorporated into the programme planning.

Monitoring and Evaluation

Any educational activity should have evaluation and assessment built into its design and implementation, which is vital for its success in all contexts. As teams are usually comprised of medical and nursing clinicians, there may be a requirement to consult with a medical educational or evaluation expert prior to commencing the activity.

A common misconception of conducting evaluation in low-resource settings is that honest feedback will not be obtained from participants due to cultural factors and potential power imbalances mentioned in the previous section. When local clinicians are reliant on visiting an NGO to provide medical services, the provision of constructive or negative feedback is potentially constrained. It has been acknowledged that poor evaluation and quality improvement practices are factors that may lead to dysfunctional partnerships in this setting.

One mechanism to achieve true evaluation is the use of anonymised feedback, with an emphasis on programme improvement rather than individual faculty assessment. Traditionally, paper-based forms are used but when these are collected and collated by the visiting team, there is the potential for identification of individuals or the perception that this may occur. Online survey apps such as Qualtrics can be used by participants on their personal devices which can improve the fidelity of collected data, and the ease of migration for analysis. One simple method of evaluation is the use of Likert scale responses with the pre- and post-course questionnaires, which should be combined with free text answers to allow the participants to add comments. A structure of asking the "most useful" and "least useful" aspects of the educational activity can provide valuable insights. Sessions that do not score highly will need to be adapted and discussion with local faculty will guide this process. Utilising these techniques in the MCHI/MCS Myanmar programme, although a high median score was obtained for sessions, there was always a large range of responses indicating honest feedback.

The visiting team faculty should also demonstrate a degree of intellectual candour during activities. Honest feedback and reflection between visiting team members will create a safe environment and promote these behaviours among participants and help to build relationships with local colleagues.

Faculty Building and Targeted Scholarships

With educational activities in LMICs, there should be a focus on the development of local faculty, who should be included in the delivery of educational content, ideally from the outset. Delivery may need to be shared initially for reasons such as relative inexperience with various SBE modalities, and unfamiliarity with course content. Concerns about hierarchy may also exist at the start of a programme. Local faculty must have access to all educational materials and should be offered development opportunities. Courses focussing on education theory and application, and research skills can be extremely beneficial, as can the provision of targeted scholarships in HIC partner institutions.

Correlation between Educational and Clinical Outcomes

The clinical impact of a SBE intervention is the real measure of success of any educational programme. There is increasing evidence in HIC settings that the application of a simulation-based mastery learning (SBML) and SBE leads to improved clinical outcomes. Changes in clinician behaviour and practice in any setting are generally multifactorial and therefore difficult to attribute to a specific educational intervention. Good data is essential and may require upskilling of local faculty in collection techniques and the use of prospective databases. The importance of these processes should be highlighted, with the understanding that this often adds to often high workloads of local clinicians.

Examples of clinical databases should be provided, including the key clinical outcome measures that need to be collected, and data points should be rationalised to facilitate their collection. Although not without potential challenges it can be achieved, as demonstrated by the change in practice and patient outcomes for the MCHI/MCS intussusception project at Yangon Children's Hospital. The project involved different aspects, including a theoretical workshop, an *in situ* SBE activity with role play in the clinical radiology department and pre- and post-implementation clinical data collection. In the post-implementation follow-up, there was a significant reduction in overall operative intervention rates: 82.5% (85/103) vs. 58.7% (44/75) vs. p = 0.006. The success for air enema reduction was 94.4% (34/36), with a recurrence rate of 5.6% (2/36).

Data may be sufficient to warrant publication, as there is significant cross-over between evaluation and research. Local ownership of data must be maintained, and co-authorship promoted. Ethics approval by all institutions must be sought.

SUMMARY

There are significant potential benefits for LMICs with the provision of educational activities; however, these must be **planned appropriately**, **be relevant to the particular setting** and **have minimal impact on the provision of local clinical services**. This is not possible without the formation and fostering of a strong partnership between the HIC and LMIC organisations, and the individuals involved. For this, there must be an acknowledgement of issues of power imbalance and hierarchy that are based on complex socio-political and economic histories. SBE modalities have demonstrated efficacy in low-resource settings, and sustainability should be at the core of any activity, whether this is a transition to educational delivery by local faculty, or capacity building in the provision of clinical services. Co-ordination of planned activities with other international organisations may be challenging but should be considered, and involvement of the local healthcare or educational institution is essential. Finally, all activities should have equity as a guiding principle.

FURTHER READING

Bogen EM, Schlachta CM, Ponsky T. White paper: Technology for surgical telementoring—SAGES project 6 technology working group. Surg Endosc. 2019;33:684–90.

Chao TE, Mandigo M, Opoku-Anane J, Maine R. Systematic review of laparoscopic surgery in low- and middle-income countries: Benefits, challenges, and strategies. Surg Endosc. 2016;30:1–10.

Cook DA, Hatala R, Brydges R, et al. Technology-enhanced simulation for health professions education: A systematic review and meta-analysis. JAMA. 2011;306:978–88.

Eichbaum QG, Adams LV, Evert J, Ho M-J, Semali IA, Schalkwyk SC van. Decolonizing global health education: Rethinking institutional partnerships and approaches. Acad Med. 2020;96:329–35.

Fergusson SJ, Sedgwick DM, Ntakiyiruta G, Ntirenganya F. The basic surgical skills course in sub-Saharan Africa: An observational study of effectiveness. World J Surg. 2018;42:930–6.

Larson CP, Plamondon KM, Dubent L, et al. The equity tool for valuing global health partnerships. Global Heal Sci Pract. 2022;10:e2100316.

Mullapudi B, Grabski D, Ameh E, et al. Estimates of number of children and adolescents without access to surgical care. Bull World Health Organ. 2019;97:254–8.

Puri L, Das J, Pai M, et al. Enhancing quality of medical care in low income and middle income countries through simulation-based initiatives: Recommendations of the simnovate global health domain group. BMJ Simul Technol Enhanc Learn. 2017;3:S15–22.

Shrime MG, Alkire BC, Grimes C, Chao TE, Poenaru D, Verguet S. Cost-effectiveness in global surgery: Pearls, pitfalls, and a checklist. World J Surg. 2017;41:1401–13.

Watters DAK, Ewing H, McCaig E. Three phases of the pacific islands project (1995–2010). Anz J Surg. 2012;82:318–24.

Weiser TG, Regenbogen SE, Thompson KD, et al. An estimation of the global volume of surgery: A modelling strategy based on available data. The Lancet. 2008;372:139–44.

Yin Mar Oo, Nataraja RM. The application of simulation-based education in low- and middle-income countries; the Myanmar experience. Semin Pediatr Surg. 2020;29:150910.

Common Problems in Remote and Rural Paediatric Surgical Practice

16

Daniel Carroll

INTRODUCTION

Over the past 20 years, attempts to rationalise and centralise care have seen services stripped out of organisations in rural and remote areas. The pace and scale of this change has accelerated over recent years. In some areas, particularly in geographically large areas, this has resulted in an increasing inequity in the provision of healthcare to certain areas and populations. Many larger organisations have sought to expand their influence into these areas by centralising services, but this has not been shown to improve patient satisfaction and fails to address important issues of cultural safety for indigenous populations.

However, there is call for optimism in some areas. There has been a pushback against the removal of services and a recognition of the importance of rural and regional specialists in Australia to try and improve healthcare access to remote and rural populations. Here in Townsville, we have tried to regain the initiative by providing in-reach services into the larger hospitals in our region. By partnering with our medical school and being actively involved in training doctors for our region, we hope we have managed to build relationships with local clinicians to allow for delivery of a comprehensive paediatric surgical service to our population.

In this chapter, we will discuss strategies for the future as well as discussing the challenges of providing comprehensive paediatric surgical care in a smaller department.

PROVIDING HEALTHCARE TO INDIGENOUS POPULATIONS

Aboriginal and Torres Strait Islander (ATSI) people experience inequalities in healthcare treatment and outcomes. Barriers to ATSI people accessing healthcare services are amplified by geographical factors. Regional and remote areas receive less healthcare funding per capita, with very remote areas receiving less than a third of the funding of major cities. People living in regional and remote areas are often

DOI: 10.1201/9781003156659-16

required to travel to metropolitan centres to access specialist services. Engagement with ATSI patients has identified a number of important areas in which healthcare for ATSI patients can be improved:

- Improved co-ordination of healthcare services
- Better communication between healthcare services and patients
- Improving trust between the service provider and improving the experience of cultural safety
- The availability of reliable, affordable and sustainable healthcare services
- Improving transport availability

In general, healthcare outcomes can best be improved by engagement with the community. We attempt to do that in our healthcare system by the employment of Indigenous Liaison Officers who play a vital role in improving our relationship with the families of our patients by ensuring their healthcare needs are met in a culturally safe environment wherever possible.

The hope for the future is that emerging elders of our first nations people here in Australia continue to train as healthcare professionals, and by returning to service their communities, we can build together a healthcare system that really begins to meet the needs of ATSI people.

The Challenge of Subspecialisation as a Generalist

Paediatric surgeons are perhaps the last of the general surgeons. The training still remains general, although many paediatric surgeons working in larger centres would see a stark difference in the variety of cases that are dealt with in our centre. Here we need to be able to manage trauma, burns, complex urology and neonatal surgery, as well as the more mundane general surgery in childhood. Increasingly subspecialisation among general surgery and adult urology colleagues means that there is a smaller pool of surgeons to call upon to provide services to paediatric patients. Trainees are no longer routinely exposed to paediatric surgery during general surgical training and sometimes have little exposure to paediatric surgery at medical school as increasingly there are more and more things to learn in the same time.

Workforce planning has often used the blunt tool of waiting lists and patient numbers to determine the number of surgeons required to operate a paediatric surgical service, but population shifts (such as occurred during COVID) can be rapid resulting in unmet need in areas that are growing rapidly. The need for future planning of departments and succession planning are self-evident but often not acted upon until a crisis occurs. Small rotas provide significant challenges for individuals in achieving a sustainable work-life balance and limit opportunities for training and achievement of continuing professional development requirements. The difficulty in recruiting locums means that unexpected or even planned leave is difficult to take without placing excessive burdens on colleagues.

There are no complete solutions to these problems, but I think the following steps have been useful in our department trying to meet these challenges:

- Regular meetings between all consultants to discuss patients and problems in the department.
- Combined operating for difficult (and/or interesting cases). This allows us to increase our experience and learn from each other as well as support each other.
- Regular MDT meetings with other healthcare professionals sharing our patients (radiology/neonatology/burns).
- Flexibility between colleagues and administration when taking leave.
- Early adoption of technologies that reduce operative workload and improve outcomes.
- Staying closely involved with other centres in Queensland with regular State-wide teaching and morbidity and mortality meetings.
- Remaining involved with teaching, training and research with opportunities with the medical school and board of paediatric surgery.

Whilst none of these measures alone can solve the problems of isolated practice and frequent on-call, they all improve engagement and support for surgeons as well providing opportunities to improve outcomes for our patients. Each of us has developed specific interests within the department and we look forward to training more paediatric surgeons (partly in the hope that we will be able to bring them into the workforce here).

Another strategy for improving outcomes for our patients is to reduce travel time for families. This 'hub and spoke' model means that our job entails frequent travel to other centres (principally Cairns/Mackay and Thursday Island [in the Torres Strait]). This can be very tiring and time-consuming, and gaps need to be made in rosters to accommodate this service. The advances in telehealth and telemedicine have reduced the requirement for travel to our patients, but the increased workload from managing patients remotely is significant. We are very reliant on the support of our colleagues in remote areas for supporting this area of practice. A joined-up approach to healthcare would greatly improve funding for these services, to reduce the burden on patients travelling for specialist healthcare services. This would require significant collaboration between many different levels of federal and state government.

Managing Uncertainty

One of the commonest problems we encounter in day-to-day practice is dealing with uncertainty in the assessment of patients who are located outside our hospital. We often have to make decisions with incomplete information where even straightforward investigations such as radiology and blood tests are not available. The medical staff in remote and rural centres are often more junior with little clinical experience to fall back on. The communication skills required to draw out a detailed clinical picture are perhaps the biggest challenge in practice. Furthermore, the decision to transfer a patient into long distances for further assessment is often met with resistance from families due to cultural or domestic problems, and from transport services in times of peak demand or when patient transport is dangerous during weather events. There is no substitute for experience in this regard, and I have often sought advice from other colleagues when decision-making is difficult.

It is often the case that we have to use all of the resources we have available, including local expertise and support from Royal Flying Doctor Service (RFDS) or retrieval doctors as well as PICU and paediatric colleagues locally and remotely to come to the best decision for the patient. The use of teleconferences to discuss patients who may need to be transferred has become a common part of my practice.

Key Messages

- Managing uncertainty is difficult in specialist practice.
- Communication and reliance on colleagues are important.

Managing Rare Conditions

A lot of patients present differently in tropical regions. We see a far greater burden of disease from infectious causes than seen in metropolitan areas. It is necessary to adjust the differential diagnosis accordingly to take into account the different spectrum of disease we see. Sepsis is much more common (often due to osteomyelitis or bacterial endocarditis and rheumatic heart disease). Some conditions are rarer (such as pyloric stenosis), whilst some are much more common (*balanitis xerotica obliterans* [BXO] and empyema). A number of conditions are not seen in other areas and, as such, are not encountered during training and are not discussed in most commonly used textbooks or other resources. In particular, conditions such as dengue fever, melioidosis and typhoid can masquerade as surgical pathologies. The involvement of paediatricians and infectious disease experts locally has been very helpful to me in transitioning from a very different environment in the UK to life in the tropics. The usefulness of regular combined consultant meetings to discuss patients cannot be overstated; this is particularly helpful in recognising and managing rare conditions.

CLIMATE CHANGE AND EXTREME WEATHER EVENTS IN THE TROPICS

Climate change is one of the biggest threats facing humanity. Even if climate change can be kept to a minimum, there is no doubt there will be a significant increase in temperature in tropical areas as well as increased risk of extreme weather events (Figure 16.1).

These have significant impact on our health today and into the future. Climate change is already impacting health, including by leading to death and illness from increasingly frequent extreme weather events, such as heatwaves, storms and floods, the disruption of food systems, increases in food-, water- and vector-borne diseases.

Furthermore, climate change is undermining many of the social determinants for good health, such as livelihoods, equality and access to healthcare and social support structures. These climate-sensitive health risks are disproportionately felt by the most vulnerable and disadvantaged, including women, children, poor communities and those with underlying health conditions.

We know from previous extreme weather events that disruption to healthcare services can be significant resulting in worse outcomes for patients in periods around these events. It often takes a significant period of time for healthcare services to return to normal and more frequent events in the future will require increased investment in areas susceptible to the effects of climate change.

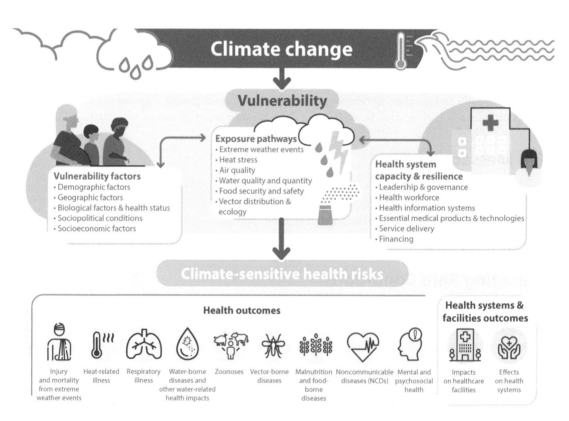

FIGURE 16.1 An overview of climate-sensitive health risks, their exposure pathways and vulnerability factors. Climate change impacts health both directly and indirectly and is strongly mediated by environmental, social and public health determinants. (From WHO Climate Change and Health.)

Maintaining Skills and Accessing Continual Professional Development (CPD)

It is an essential part of good clinical practice to maintain and update skills. This is a particular challenge for surgeons working in a geographically isolated position. Although we are part of mainland Australia, transport options to attend meetings and to operate with colleagues are limited. Travel time also limits our availability to attend meetings and to remain involved with other colleagues. The transition of meetings to an online format as a response to the COVID pandemic has been a blessing in disguise for us here in North Queensland. The ability to access and actively participate in meetings without the need for travel has been hugely beneficial. The need to maintain skills and to update practice is perhaps more relevant to those working in a more isolated practice and these needs should be accounted for when planning a sustainable department with improved access to professional development leave and enhanced study leave budgets. Such requirements are not met at the moment and without change from State and Federal governments to support regional surgeons my expectation is that it will become increasingly difficult to maintain high-quality service outside of major metropolitan areas and health inequity will rise.

THE FUTURE

The only certainty is that the future will hold significant change. The pace of change in society and medicine has increased over recent decades and this will no doubt continue. Despite the challenges to practice in remote and regional areas, it remains a hugely rewarding area to practice in. The rise of populations in the tropics will require a shift in skills and training to meet demand. We will no doubt lag behind the clinical need in these areas, but a shift in thinking among politicians and healthcare administrators will hopefully result in fundamental changes in training and methods of healthcare delivery to meet the demands of our population. I feel certain that enhanced telemedicine has a huge role to play in our region. Advances in technology will hopefully reduce the requirement for surgery by diagnosing and treating diseases earlier and more effectively. Artificial Intelligence solutions have already shown great promise and advances in computer technology will undoubtedly play a part in improving healthcare outcomes in paediatric surgery. Ultimately the greatest hope for the future is the next generation of paediatric surgeons and medical students. Hopefully by engaging with ATSI communities, we will continue to see rising numbers of medical school graduates particularly from universities such as ours who aspire to 'close the gap' for educational opportunity and achievement.

"The future belongs to those who believe in the beauty of their dreams."

—Eleanor Roosevelt

FURTHER READING

Atiyeh BS, Gunn SW, Hayek SN. Provision of essential surgery in remote and rural areas of developed as well as low and middle income countries. Int J Surg. 2010;8(8):581–5.

Fraser S, Grant J, Mackean T, Hunter K, Holland AJA, Clapham K, Teague WJ, Ivers RQ. Burn injury models of care: A review of quality and cultural safety for care of indigenous children. Burns. 2018 May;44(3):665–77.

Watts N, et al. The 2020 report of the Lancet countdown on health and climate change: Responding to converging crises. Lancet. 2021 January;397(10269):129–70.

Index

Note: Locators in *italics* represent figures and **bold** indicates tables in the text.